Coming Undone

Coming Undone

A Memoir

Terri White

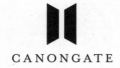

CANONGATE

Caution: this book contains references to sexual and other physical abuse, self-harm, addiction and suicidal ideation.

First published in Great Britain in 2020
by Canongate Books Ltd, 14 High Street, Edinburgh EH1 1TE

canonongate.co.uk

2

British Library Cataloguing-in-Publication Data
A catalogue record for this book is available on
request from the British Library

ISBN 978 1 78689 678 0

Typeset in Garamond MT Std 12.5/16 pt by
Palimpsest Book Production Ltd, Falkirk, Stirlingshire

Printed and bound in Great Britain by Clays Ltd, Elcograf S.p.A.

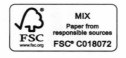

For Margaret Noreen Carter.
And all the girls who fear they're forever lost.

CHAPTER 1

In my right hand is a transparent bag holding my clothes, basic toiletries and loose items of make-up. I step towards the automatic doors, which, sensing the movement, open with a whoosh: curtains announcing the matinee performance. I move forwards one small step, a second, and I'm through them, out on the street. I stand entirely still, close my eyes, breathe in, hold for two beats and then open my eyes wide and allow the world outside in.

Beeeeeeeeeep.

Beeeeeeeeeeeeeeeppppppppp.

A yellow cab speeds past, horn blaring at a weaving cyclist who narrowly misses bouncing off its front bumper. A woman in a beige woollen skirt suit with a thin pink trim, short rigid curls and a face worn tight, bends down to scoop up her small white dog's neatly laid shit with a tinted plastic bag, turned inside out and worn over her fingers and thumb. The bag might be scented, probably is, but I can't isolate and identify that smell over the other smells writhing on top of each other, vying for attention. The odours of an average New York City street on an average spring day: garbage, coffee, noodles, piss, hotdogs, burnt sugar, beer, bagels. Sweet, bitter, soft, strong and sharp. The smells that become tastes when they travel up into your nose and down through your throat.

The grey, uneven patchwork pavement shakes, sizzles and bakes beneath my feet. I look from left to right, down at the concrete and up at the sky, or what's visible of it between the towering buildings on this block. Wisps of white clouds scatter across an otherwise blemish-free blue sky; the sun blazes, burns bright. Tucked under my left arm are the flowers I was sent with love five days ago, by one of the handful of people who know the truth about where I've been. I had insisted on carrying them out with me, hand tight around the base of the basket, even though the flowers, the yellow and white daisies that had brought sunshine into the green ward, died yesterday. The heads are bowed and broken and brown, the soil flaky and cracked. I pull them closer. I flag a taxi with the hand holding the bag, my belongings held aloft and bared. I step down off the kerb, open the door, climb in the back and – just like that – I slide back into my life.

'Avenue D and Third,' I say to the driver.

I'm going back to my apartment in the East Village. My corner was once one of the very worst corners, the darkest corner of Manhattan's drugs and crime-controlled no-go area. It's now home to people like me, who push rental prices up and up, encouraging a Starbucks to open just two and a half blocks away.

Arriving home, I check my mailbox, which is over-flowing, walk up the three flights of stairs and open the grey front door to my apartment, expecting resistance on the other side. Thirteen days ago, it was a wreck; more specifically the wreckage of a life in bits. The sink was stacked with dirty dishes, the worktops covered with take-out cartons and empty bottles. In the living room a carpet of crunched-up beer cans, wine bottles rolling on their sides, the prongs of plastic forks sticking in my foot every time I tiptoed to the bathroom, which was covered in damp towels, dirty clothes. In the bedroom, there were more discarded clothes, twisted stained sheets, fallen single shoes and bobby pins scattered like tiny traps across the bed and floor.

I feel both a rush of gratitude and a wave of shame crash into my chest as I walk into a transformed apart-ment. I don't allow myself to think of my friend's reaction when she came in, the door proving unyielding at first, after I gave her my keys to pick up some clothes. The message she will inevitably have shared, flying from Manhattan to Brooklyn and back again: *did you all know about the mess? About how bad things were? Should we clean it? She can't return to that, surely?*

I picture her, picking up the discarded pills, one by one. The survivors that were last seen falling from my mouth, sticking underfoot and skidding into dark corners. The breadcrumb trail that didn't lead me out of the woods, but was proof that I had been deep, deep in there, lost among the trees.

I drop my bag by the door, put my dead flowers down on the desk. A curled, crisp leaf lands by my feet. I look out of the window, hear sirens ringing out on the streets below. I become cold with fear, unable to move. *Are they coming for me?*

CHAPTER 2

Eight days earlier.

'Hi! Um, I think there's been a mistake,' I say casually, with what I hope is an easy smile, high on the smallest glimmer of hope. There's a noise, meant to pass as a light laugh, but which falls out of my throat somewhere between a hacking cough and a muffled squeal. The thick-bodied, heavy-eyed doctor stares an inch or so over my left shoulder and shakes his head. The forms I absolutely must sign are pushed towards me, curled up in his hand. He's already filled his part in.

'It'll be more difficult for you if you refuse. *This* will all take longer,' he says, gesturing around the room.

He should have made it home already, long before the sun outside turned orange and the sky beneath it went from blue to grey to black. His hair, brown and floppy – not unlike that of the boy who'd been my first frenzied obsession back in junior school – grazes the lids of his eyes as he blinks slowly, looks away, over my head, anywhere but at me. I try to make contact, convinced that once we lock eyes he'll see the truth, as opposed to what presumably currently looks like manic terror, madness given voice. Can't both be real? Both *are* real, to me, right now.

My fingers, freed after being strapped to the stretcher under blankets in the ambulance that conveyed me here, move up inside the sticky brown beehive pinned to my head. A habit which only a few – and certainly not this man, a stranger, yet one who already has such power – know to read as fear, my nerves prickling, rising, pressing against, needling my skin. I have a hospital bracelet on my left wrist, bearing a bleached-out picture of me. I know it's me but I don't recognise the face that stares back. The patterned hospital gown doesn't quite reach my elbows but does reach past my knees; it's tied at the back with three ties. The thin cotton socks from the previous hospital are still on my feet, which turn inwards as I stand, trying to think fast, not fast enough.

I make a small concession and take the forms and the pen, hands shaking, see the X where my signature is meant to go, the blank spot for my name. I don't bring pen to paper. Instead I say, 'Thanks! But I really want to talk to somebody. You know, now.' I'm attempting a tricky balance between begging and assertiveness.

He looks at me finally, confused by the words I've just said.

'Well,' I say, in answer to the question he hasn't asked yet, 'about going home today. I just need to talk to someone quickly. It won't take long. I've been in the other hospital for five days and want to arrange my discharge.'

I try to keep the panic out of my mouth and the edge out of my words. I've been planning this speech all the way over in the ambulance, not to mention for the last five and a half days and five nights I've been in another bed waiting for this one. The precise words and how they rise and fall and land in his ears. I can't blow it now. He must see how sane I am. I try to ignore the mounting alarm, regulate every beat and breath as I realise that I only have seconds, not even minutes, to show him, convince him, make him understand who I am and how all of this is the most terrible of mistakes. I don't belong here. Surely he can see that. Surely anyone could. I'm not entirely sure what a crazy person is supposed to look like, but I'm pretty sure it's not this; it's not me.

A small, bemused shake of his head and his stare disconnects, a light, my hope extinguished. 'I've been waiting for you to arrive. I should have left already,' he says. 'There's no one here to talk about it now. We can talk about it tomorrow, properly, but for now, you just need to sign. You can't just go home.'

The spit of his impatience sticks to me, even as his gaze doesn't leave the heavy air by my ear, where his eyes have moved once more. I think about the wife who pushed the golden band onto the second finger of his left hand, of their children, the calls to let him know that yes, they are still waiting for him and why hasn't he left yet? The dinner bubbling in the oven, getting hard and losing flavour with each minute I delay him further. Around the table later, water glasses filled, ice melted, he'll say how sorry he is, that the latest mad girl was admitted super late and he was the only one who could stay and she started asking to leave and he knows it's only twelve hours until he has to be back there and he's already said he's sorry.

I start to read or, more specifically, push my eyes backwards and forwards, left and right across the page, slowly, hoping to buy even just a small fistful of time to think. I need it all to stop so I can just fucking think, press pause for a minute, make the world, this reality, stop. I sit on the bed and try to work it all out, so that when I press play again it will all be fixed and I won't be scared.

But I am scared. Terrified. Because right now, none of this is going how I'd planned. I'd run this scenario in my head a hundred times or more and in each story, each sequence of events, I'm released back onto the city streets down below, relieved and, most importantly, free. Once I'm safely home, I put all of this down to a momentary silly slip, followed by an official overreaction, and within a few hours I'm eating alone in the bar of a restaurant, my third martini kicking against the back of my throat – empty and open.

The story in my brain sends the signal to my mouth and it floods with water, my tongue lapping against the wet waves. My mind wanders to smoky Irish whiskies warmed in the glass, a crisp, precise lager that dances and bubbles across my tongue, a wine that takes me to the Andalusian mountains and beyond. The shadow of my senses forms a solid shape, takes flight and moves just beyond my touch, my taste, my smell. The doctor sighs once more, harder and heavier this time, and all of the moisture is sucked out of my mouth.

I lick my lips, shake my head a little and focus, continuing to read, though none of the words and sentences are working their way through my eyes into my brain and becoming substance, becoming fact. They sit, instead, just inside my eyeballs, very still, intact but immovable, unknowable.

Though I don't know what it says, I do know what it means. It means that my plan didn't work. The one that was going to see me walk straight out of here, only minutes after walking straight in. An hour tops. We were meant to talk, laugh a little, shake hands, then off I'd go, plastic bag containing all my belongings swinging in one hand.

But now, the sun's pretty much set on Thursday and I know in this moment that I'm now facing the weekend in here, at least. I can't remember if he says this or if I just know it, instinctively, but it's a fact. It could, in total, be days, weeks or even months: it definitely won't be hours.

I look at his brown lace-up shoes, beige chinos, preppy blue starched shirt and black fleece with a high zip that must tickle his chin when he looks down at the floor, at his feet, which I imagine he does a lot. He isn't like me. Or rather, I'm not like him. He doesn't see who I am and certainly won't in the window of time we have together tonight.

My stomach is in my socks – I don't have shoes – as I submit, pressing the pen against the paper and pulling until my name, or a version of it, appears. I want to throw up but I smile, tighter now, and rest one hand on my belly in a futile attempt to stop it leaping and twisting with the knowledge and awareness of what I've just signed on for. I don't know specifically what awaits me in the coming days or weeks, but I do know that this is the most dire, desperate situation I've ever found myself in. And I've been in a few. I've never felt more trapped; I've never been more trapped.

The reality of it travels through my body like urgent news down a wire – pins and needles sprinkle into my fingertips where they burst, tiny fireworks under my nails. Every cliché is coming alive in my body: the room spins; my head swims; I lose feeling in my ankles, my hands; everything out of my immediate eyesight is fizzy and fuzzy and distorted. The room goes cold, while heat floods my head. I can't believe I'm still standing – I have to touch the desk to my left, just to make sure, in fact, that I am.

The part of me that I've only ever got a weak hold on pulls and tugs before breaking off and floating up to the ceiling; she squats in the darkness of the corner, staring at the top of both of our heads. It occurs to me for a second that I might have died and this might be death, the afterlife, or at least the life after. Every feeling in every inch of my body is alien, obscure, beyond my understanding. What other explanation is there?

I gather enough of my mind and my body to ask: 'So how long will I need to be here?' as I hand him back the pen and papers, now signed so he can leave. Which he starts to do immediately, shuffling past me as he says, 'We don't know. It's impossible to say. You'll be able to talk to someone about all of that soon.' And with that he's gone, out of the door. The door to the place that I've now agreed to call home, so the doctor can return to his.

It's time to survive. I call her down from the ceiling and send her back into my body. This is how I'll make it through: I'll do what I'm told, what I must. What day is it? Thursday. OK. Can it really have been just Saturday that I was told in no uncertain terms that no, I couldn't go home? It was. How many more days until I could go home? At least three. Probably more. I've survived almost six; I can take more. How can I get out? I need somebody to see, or at least agree I don't belong here. I mean, I *don't* belong here. I'm sure everyone says this. But I don't, truly. I can't; I just can't. And if the doctor can't see that, which, I'm guessing by his attitude he either can't or won't, I need to find the person who will. I will be the good little girl, barely causing an eyebrow to raise, while I tick off each day and wait, quietly. I'm not free, but the only way to become so again is to submit, willingly, with a closed throat.

Now it's just me and the male nurse, who's been standing silently watching our entire exchange. It's not the first time he's witnessed this, clearly. He first takes my obs – blood pressure, temperature and pulse rate – the three-times-a-day ritual to measure my vital signs that I'll come to know well. He then picks up and empties my plastic bag, the one that had transported my belongings from the hospital downtown. He sorts through them methodically, a sharpened pencil in one hand, itemising them, line by line: laptop, clothes, shoes, toiletries, make-up. Almost everything is a danger to me, because I'm officially a danger to me. I keep the make-up that doesn't have sharp edges or is encased in glass: my lipstick, eyeliner, mascara. I keep a notebook and a pencil; he takes my laptop. I haven't had my phone since the night this all started. I can't have my shoes with laces, even though each lace – which couldn't be more than twelve inches long – would only really make a noose suitable for a mouse.

He starts to fold up my clothes. 'Wait,' I say. 'I need to take something to wear.' As is becoming routine, he shakes his head: I can't have my clothes yet. Not for the first day or two. He doesn't say why, though the next day another patient tells me I 'have to earn them'. No one from the hospital staff has said this is the case, but these words hit me. Earn my *own* clothes, the right not to have my backside hanging out. It feels like punishment. Like a marking of those newly mad or at least newly declared mad: the shuffling in socks and gaping gowns making you look as unkempt and loose, as wild, as lacking in civility and humanity as you feel. And with it comes a new feeling: shame. Like being painted with a thick brush from the ends of the hairs on your toes to the ends of the hair on your head.

The humiliation stirs a fist of anger within me. But I don't say anything; I don't put kindling against the flame and allow it to burn bigger. I just nod. Smile. My confiscated belongings are taken to a storage room at the end of the corridor, to sit in their plastic bag in a box, next to a row of other plastic bags in boxes. If I want anything from it, I'm to ask and they will supervise me using whatever it is I need. But they ask that people don't do that unless it's absolutely necessary. I wonder what necessary really means. And how many seconds you'd have to smash the mirror and take the thickest of the jagged shards to the thinnest part of your throat before anyone noticed or bothered to try and stop you.

He gestures to my hair, to the bobby pins keeping my beehive erect. 'No, no, no,' I say, a little too quickly, suddenly acutely aware of the speed, emphasis, intonation and volume of what I say. Every word. I push the ends of my fingers into my palm to cause me to pause, allow a beat and then say, calmly: 'They're not sharp, honestly, they're just hair grips.' He looks confused. 'Um, bobby pins. Please, let me keep them. Look, touch one.' I pull one out of my hair to show him, handing it over, showing him how to run his finger over the cold, round, perfectly harmless edge. He nods, hands it back and I let out a deep sigh of relief. In truth, it's probably not entirely harmless. I almost certainly could do *something* to my body with it. With enough force, will, pressure and impact. But right now, my mind isn't on gutting myself with a hair grip, but on retaining what is left of my dignity, however tiny the pieces I'm gathering in my palm. As of this moment, my hair, my beehive, the grips holding it all in place, is all I have. I can't lose it now, the scraps of me.

He starts to leave, trailing my plastic bag behind him on the floor before pausing. 'There are no closed doors in here. They must be kept open.' I nod again. Smile again. And then it's just me. I sit on the bed, salt on my tongue, swallowing the taste of vomit as it rises to graze the back of my throat. It burns. My eyes burn. My belly burns. The fire fills me, quietly.

I take my first proper look around the room. I see that my room is for two patients, though the second bed hasn't yet been slept in and the very few belongings I've been allowed to keep are the only ones in the room. There are two desks, two chairs, two thin beds, with white sheets and green blankets tucked in tightly, two glaring strip-lights above. A bathroom with a shower, the plastic yellow cubicle built into the corner of the room, a sink, a mirror and a toilet. I'm so relieved that there's no one else in the room to witness me stripped back and full of terror. I don't know if I'll be joined by a roommate or when. As I do in every room, scared of who or what will come through the door, I take the bed closest to the window.

Looking up, I see the looming towers that make the shape of New York, the city glimmering and winking through the black wire mesh pulled tight across the window. Every window down the farthest wall is covered in the same black wire mesh. Everything viewed through it has a grey, used-up look. Like it's been left out in the sun, the colour burned off the top after years of brutal exposure.

We're up eight floors high. I think of ripping the mesh open with my fingers and trying to smash through the window with my balled fists. But I don't. I breathe, consider the new land ahead. Uncharted territory. I'm thirty-four years old and now, I suppose, finally, officially mad.

I was seven the first time I went mad, I think. Six? Maybe it wasn't actually the first time. But it was the first time that I remember, remember feeling it, hearing it, being it. The breeze in my belly becoming a squall, picking up scraps that rattled out a new, distorted tune on my ribs. I'd clambered out of the bedroom window of our council house, a window which would come to be tied tightly shut with white shoelaces, to keep me in. Balancing on the ledge, I knew absolutely that I wouldn't fly, that I would fall. My despair was quieted just for a moment by the thought of my body dropping through the air like a stone, hitting the ground. I remember how

15

the cold air soothed my cheek as I looked out over the houses and gardens that surrounded us. I didn't look at the ground directly below but knew it was there, could see my body spreadeagled, face-down on the grass, limbs at extraordinary, impossible angles.

No one tells you how to be mad when you're six, when you're seven; no one tells you what it looks like, sounds like, feels like. But no one tells you how not to be, either. Or why you shouldn't be. I would sneak biros from the dresser drawer, snap them in half and pull the splintered plastic edges down my arms. I watched myself crying in the mirror while 10cc tried to drown out the kids playing outside. They were still too loud. It had been coming a while, even then. How *can* it have been coming a while? At six, at seven? The pain, the burden, the weight already felt like too much to bear. My slight shoulders buckled and corrected, while I struggled to stay on two feet.

So, it was no great surprise, really, that I ended up on that ledge. Or that twenty-seven years on, and three thousand miles away, I would end up on another. The wire across the windows replacing the shoelaces that kept me safe when I tried to fall, when I believed I could, would. The pain of the past, shaped and shrouded in black, shaking off the soil I'd buried it under, comes crawling towards me, moaning as it drags and pulls itself along. It inches through the door here on the psych ward and I feel it pulling at my hair, let it loosen the pins I'd just fought desperately to keep.

I stand at the window, looking at the fluorescent-lit bricks of the building opposite, the outline of the city as it roars and settles. I dream of flying, of being, for the very first time, free – even while all I can hear is the ground rushing towards me.

CHAPTER 3

Here's where it begins. Or rather, here's where it ends. Six nights prior, in a charmless midtown sports bar, ceiling lights down low, blue LED strip-lights plotting the exact dimensions of the room. Three of the walls are decorated with framed pictures of the city through the ages and neon bar signs depicting bubbles running down the outside of a jauntily angled beer glass, bright green lucky clovers tucked into the corner of the glowing tube.

I'm here at the invitation of a man I know from back home in England, though barely. He suggested drinks as a guise to ask me for a job. I said yes so I could drink with an excuse and company. As the third pint empties into my throat and the bottom of the glass hits the table, he leaves, to get back to his wife. I stay drinking, without excuse, without company and without question. After three drinks I need none.

As I swallow more, the crowd blurs and fizzes and rattles around me. I look up and it reaches the very edges of the room: four deep at the bar, every red plastic stool smothered in damp skin and cloth. Everyone is represented: office workers, restaurant servers, shop assistants, management execs, bartenders from other bars down the block. Ice hockey is on every single television screen that papers the wall: the clashing and crashing of sticks and bones blares out in waves, sliced through with screams and whoops from the room with increasing frequency. No time passes; hours disappear, and I look up again and the people have disappeared, dissolving into the air around me. I count the people on one hand, maybe the beginnings of two. Those of us who stayed beyond the acceptable post-work drinking hours and were now into our time. Where conversation isn't the point. Drinking is. It's the only point.

Then, now, nothing.

Blackouts are a weekly, daily visitor by then. I no longer wait to be seduced; I chase, hunt them down hungrily, teeth, tongue bared. Wine follows whisky follows anything wet and strong until the plug is kicked clean out of the base of my brain. I close my eyes and enjoy the slide, the floor taking off my face.

Now, then, eyes open. I'm naked in my own bed, blotchy limbs tangled up in stained black sheets. I squint, flinch in the glare of the sunlight snaking through the bars on the window of my third-floor walk-up. My fists closed tight, I'm spreadeagled on the mattress. I'm holding something so hard my fingers have gone white. I uncurl first the left, then the right, and see an orange pill bottle tucked in each. Both are empty; they were full before, a doctor's order to take one of each a day ignored, not for the first time. Patting myself down, I find a few of the bright blue tablets stuck to my hot skin: jammed against my spine, slipped behind my ear, tucked inside the fold of my damp knee. I pluck them off one by one, put one wobbly foot on the floor and clutch the corner of the mattress to steady me, momentarily. Three more pills scatter beneath my toes, running far and wide in their bid for escape. Apart from the half-handful of plucky desperate deserters, I've swallowed down everything in those two bottles, though not a single memory of a gulp remains in my mind, no matter how much I rummage.

I'm still breathing, still alive, but will I die today? Tonight? When I next sleep? I'm afraid, suddenly. The urge to vomit is overwhelming and I buckle, my body folding in half at the waist under the sheer force of a heave, my mouth filling with water. I spit it out into my palm before scrunching my hand into a fist; bubbles peek and pop through the gap where my knuckles join. It begins to creep up on me. Somehow, perhaps surprisingly, the thought of dying slowly, painfully, while sobering up terrifies me more than anything else at that moment – including surviving – and I heave, bend, baulk and spit again. My ankles shake and I struggle to stay standing without the wall to hold me.

Two days earlier, my eyes had opened for the first time to fists full of bottles. But that time, they had kept their contents. By my best guess, my suicidal bent was foiled by a mixture of child-protection caps and unconsciousness. Once I'd realised what I'd almost done, I simply swallowed an extra morning Xanax and put the Prozac and mood stabilisers back on my bedside table where I'd taken them from the night before.

Waking clutching pill bottles like flares wasn't the first sign that something was, is, wrong. This low, when it came several weeks ago, had been quick and sticky. But that day, like every day, I'd climbed into my dusty pink shower and stood with my body under the water until the skin over it turned scarlet. At pains, as usual, to stand with my hair kept out, to avoid the panic that overwhelmed me when water went over my head, in my eyes, filled my mouth. Then I patted myself with a towel briefly, pulled clothes from the floor over my damp arms and legs, poured drops into my eyeballs, painted my face bright, pinned my hair up higher and higher, tighter and tighter, and walked out of the door with as straight a back as I could manage. I walked, I smiled, I ate, I worked, I breathed in, I breathed out, I drank, I blacked out. Again, again, again, again, again.

The weeks before this one were just days and nights of sharp, paralysing fragments of pain. Memories incomplete and scattered in different corners of my brain, some beyond recovery. Most nights were missing, as were some days. The minutes and hours before a blackout and the minutes and hours when emerging from one spent googling methods of suicide:

'Painless suicide'
'Hanging yourself + how to'
'Sleeping pills + number to die'
'How to make a noose'
'Slit wrists + how deep + death'
'Instant death + hanging + height'

The previous Sunday, I'd blinked awake to find myself at the intersection of a street in the West Village, the green man walking flashing in my eyeline. My feet took me to the sidewalk outside a church, its roof rising up into the deepest blue sky. A priest on the steps, white robes glowing and swaying, beckoning me in. I'd read somewhere that priests could spot those truly in trouble, in real mortal danger, their souls set to be lost without a great, selfless intervention. Even in a crowd of thousands, their pain and peril marks them out, the swarm of black that shifts over their shape as they move. I walked towards him slowly, up the steps. He looked right through me as I passed, not noticing the screams bouncing around inside my mind.

Was I really here?
Could he see me?
Could he see the danger?
The ledge I was on?
Please see me.
Help me.
Please.
Father.

Inside, people swayed and sang, hands held aloft, trying to touch God and bring Him into them. I gripped the seat in front, my hands strangling wood. I sobbed, choked, offered up something like a prayer, or at least a plea, to whoever could hear me. I would do anything. I would become His servant. I would forsake everything if He would help me, if someone, *anyone*, would help me.

I stared desperately, helplessly, at the priest, as he showered us with a sermon in the shadow of a crucifix. He didn't look at me once. The hell burned through me and made me disappear, here, in His house. I would never be saved.

Now, on this Saturday morning, my options are even more limited than they were that day. Driven by cold fear, I decide that I have no choice but to go to the emergency room. I throw on the nearest clothes I find on the floor, straighten up my hair, swill water around in my mouth and head out of the apartment. I walk to the corner two streets away and hail a yellow taxi with hands covered in dried spit. We speed along and I press my hands against the cab window, straining towards the bright, beautiful sunshine-filled sky.

'Why did you do that?' the admissions nurse in the ER demands as I stand by her desk, crying, heaving. I shake my head, splattering her paperwork with tears as I do. She stares, unmoved. She's the first of several people to ask me the same obvious, yet impossible question when I say I believe I have taken two bottles of pills. She glances down at the wet patches on the paper in front of her and looks away again.

'I need your insurance card,' she says flatly. I slide it over the desk and she takes a photograph with a camera I can't look directly at.

I'm taken through to the emergency room, not realising that I am voluntarily walking into a room I wouldn't be able to walk out of again. 'Why did you do that?' asks the second nurse. It becomes more of a complaint, an exasperation, than a question. I shake my head, cry again. I'm given a hospital gown to change into and socks.

The air is tight and fat and hot as a man screams complaints I can't understand from behind a half-drawn curtain. A single shoe lies on the floor next to another man, shirtless, in bloodied jeans, handcuffed to the bed, spitting. A prison officer sits and keeps watch on a prisoner being treated in the hospital from a plastic chair nearby. Metal clanks against metal as the prisoner hollers and thrashes and kicks. I put my hands over my ears to quieten the screaming, the sound of desperation and pain that I can't bear to hear.

I'm on a stretcher by the nurses' station, my sobs giving rhythm, a pulse, to the room, which spins. A nurse all in white, with a thick Eastern European accent, leans over my body and takes my arms. She has short, spiky blonde hair. I think about touching it, half move my hand into the expanse between us, and then pull it back again.

'Why did you do this?' she pleads. 'I'm not judging you. I don't know what your problems are. But this is never the answer. Tomorrow is always better.'

I cry, harder now. She continues, urging me to let God into my heart, and her empathy cuts me open and everything I feel pours out. The machines attached to me beep a tune I don't recognise as the room turns white and then black and then white and then black. People walk past, bodies grazing the stretcher as they peer at the crying, vomiting woman.

Then I'm moved into a small cubicle, given some privacy by curtains. My knees press against the white wall, which is scuffed and smeared. I lie there and the doctors pass in a group every hour on the hour – new eyes, same look, same mantra:

'Terri White, thirty-four, overdose while drinking.'

They sing the same song, each time with the same tone, the same intonation. *Te-rri-White-over-dose-while-drink-ing.* I sing along; sometimes they're there to be the chorus, other times I hold the solo alone. I look out and meet their eyes, enjoying the flinch as they look directly at my hard, stained face. I smile at some of them, head swaying to and fro as they break my gaze as soon as they can, a flash of horror touching the corners of their mouths.

My cubicle mate, just half an arm away, is an elderly woman in a patterned headscarf who burps, coughs and hacks, her ribs revealed on every breath she sucks in. Every breath looks like it may be her last.

The young mousy-haired doctor who appears by my bed – 'I'm looking for the overdose lady' – pushes wire-rimmed glasses up her nose as she asks:

'Why did you do this, Miss White?'

'Well, presumably I wanted to die,' I say.

I actually want to admit that I can't say for sure. I remember desire: the desire not to be here, simply not to be anywhere. Not so much a lust for death as a lust for nothing at all. A hunger, a need to be filled with nothing. And the quickest way to get that, to be that, was to die. Could she not understand that?

I have never been afraid of dying. But the thought that I could, would, live hundreds, even thousands of days in the same pain I'd spent the hundreds, thousands of days prior to this one in, terrified me. And in truth, so many of life's choices are simply the triumph of one kind of fear over another. But I don't say any of this, can't find the words, can't make my tongue curl and roll and dart.

'But have you wanted to die?'

Yes?

'Before, in your life?'

Yes. Of course.

'Did you want to die then?'

When?

'Last night.'

I don't know. I can't really remember. I presume so.

'Do you want to die now?'

What, right now?

'Yes.'

Well, yes.

Because right then, I do. I really do.

Then more questions, a new stranger, who I can only see the outline of: long hair, slim shoulders, thin arms. She says she needs to tick or not tick the boxes that sit on her piece of paper in a list.

'Were you trying to kill yourself?'

As I've said: yes. I presume I was.

'Do you have a history of self-harm?'

Yes.

'Have you tried to harm yourself before?'

Yes.

'How many times?'

Many.

'When?'

Often.

'Recently?'

Yes.

'Do you have thoughts of harming other people?'

No, only myself.

'Do you want to be dead?'

Yes, right now, I do.

I answer, slurring my words. The room still swings and sways. Everything lurches. I lurch. I remember most of it, but possibly not all of it. I'm not sure whether I get it all right. Did I tell her of the razor blades I used to open up my thighs with? The skin I sliced through on my arm last year, right through the fat and tissue, that's still not healed? Of the time, twelve years ago,

27

when three firemen took an axe to my front door? I can't remember.

I'm so away from myself, my mind, my good sense, that it doesn't occur to me to lie. I'm convinced that she can see straight into my heart, straight into my truth. She knows what I've done: of the booze and bleeding and pills. The dreams of rope and razors.

Hours pass, the doctor returns, an apparition with a frown. What she says doesn't make much sense the first time.

'The combination of pills you've taken doesn't normally kill you, as an overdose, actually,' she says, underlining my accidental failure. 'But we need you to stay in for observation. Because it can, sometimes, cause arrhythmia and sudden death, some hours later.'

I weigh up what she's saying. Consider it, figuring we're talking a few hours, tops.

'OK. But I can go home then, yes?'

A quick calculation reassures me that I'd be out for Sunday brunch, a solo topping-up occasion, and then work as normal on Monday. There'll barely be a dent in my normal life, my normal schedule. Things will go back to as they were. As they are. Whatever that is.

'Well, the cardiac observation is for twenty-four hours. But then, when a bed is available, you'll be transferred to the psychiatric ward.' Do I laugh? I think I might laugh. She pauses, frowns, harder now.

'We cannot let you go,' she says slowly, while looking at me like I've taken leave of any senses I have remaining.

I let out a choked cry, a sound I can't place or identify coming from the back of my throat. I'm shaking my head.

'No! No: it was an accident. There's no need.'

'You said you wanted to die, Miss White.'

'I didn't know what I was saying. I feel better now. It was an accident. It's so silly! I just want to go home.'

'You can't. You're not. You won't. The psychiatric team have made the decision.'

'Well, I'll sign myself out and take full responsibility. You can't stop me.' I try to stand.

She steps forwards. 'We can and we will.'

My throat tightens.

'What?'

My voice breaks.

'Legally, we can and will be holding you for a minimum of seventy-two hours.'

She explains that the psychiatric ward is fit to burst. That the seventy-two hours can't begin until I arrive in the ward, under specialised care. She can't tell me how long I'll be waiting. But, for now, and until then, I'd be on twenty-four-hour, one-on-one observation.

I open and close my mouth noiselessly. I think about the goldfish I had as a kid that I would take out of its bowl and pop on the silver corrugated drain by the sink, fascinated by its fight for life. How helpless, desperate and wild-eyed it looked in the face of death. Right at that moment, clutching the wall, cold and hard and rigid under my grasp, I wish I had died. I feel like I am dead. This can't be life. This can't be my life. I won't survive it.

29

The doctor writes as I continue to gasp and gulp. Then the Suicide Preventer appears: the soft-faced woman whose job it is to ensure I don't try again. The first woman in a long line of women. She arrives silently, takes her seat by the curtain, picks up the notepad and watches, constantly, writes, constantly. She looks on as I cry, close my eyes tight.

She's small and old and frail. I think of how tiny she looks. How fragile. I could overpower her. I have to get out of here and she's the only thing between me and the world, between me and freedom. I don't want to hurt her. I won't. But I want desperately to run. To say I need the toilet and then just keep walking, a half-pace quicker and quicker until I'm breaking into a run and smashing through these walls until I'm out on the street, feet pounding the sidewalk.

But even as my mind whirs and plots, I know that they know where I live, where I work, what my life looks like. I filled in too many forms. They will hunt me down and scoop me back up before I can enjoy the true taste of freedom. Things may, unbelievably, get even worse.

Hours pass, the sick sinks even further into my gums. I'm silent and still, eyes laser-focused on the wall. When I eventually do need to go to the toilet, I stand up. Start to walk. She follows me, just a couple of steps behind. When we get to the door of the disabled bathroom, I turn to face her.

'Can you wait outside, please?'

'I'm sorry, no.' She shakes her head sadly. 'Everywhere

you go, I go.' A pause as she waits for the penny to descend. 'Everywhere.'

'But I really want my privacy,' I plead. 'Please.'

She shakes her head and writes down some words I can't see on the sheet of paper she's still carrying with her. She lays the pencil to rest.

'No. Let's go.'

I open the door and we walk in together. My feet fight to run, twitch against the fabric of their socks. She locks the door and stands facing me. There's a small square mirror above the sink and as I turn to face her, I glance at my unrecognisable face, now pink, shiny and swollen, distorted like a party balloon.

I lift my gown, squat and sit on the toilet seat. I see the red emergency cord hanging down just an inch to my right. I want to pull it. I want it to set me free. Rip a hole in the ceiling that I can fly through, taking off the roof with me. But I stay with my feet on the ground, against white tiles. I open my bladder and pee.

Pssssssssst.

My pee turns the water in the bowl bright yellow. The seconds pass.

Pssstttttttttttttttttt.

The red from my chest climbs up my throat like ivy and up over my face. I look at my Suicide Preventer and she meets my eyes, holds my gaze. I'm humiliated. I'm newly fucking furious.

As I sit with my thighs spread, the dark hair between them exposed while I lock eyes with a stranger, I'm aware of how desperate my situation is. How alone I am. I have no phone, no laptop, no numbers and no way of letting anyone know where I am. How would I raise the alarm? And if I did, who could help me, who *would* help me?

New York, a city in which I have always felt insignificant, small, a nothing, has swallowed me whole, without care. And there's no indication when, or if, it will bother spitting me back out.

CHAPTER 4

I'm back in my cubicle, wearing a hospital gown, no underwear, with a blanket draped loosely over me. I clasp it between my legs tightly, seeking any comfort I can get. I'm waiting for my 'transport' to the cardiac ward. I wait and wait and don't know how many hours pass as I face the wall, the colour sucked out of my entire body. My chest spasms, contracts, expands, shrinks, flexes, tightens until I think it's going to split wide open.

I trace scratches on the wall – the cracks, the point at which the paint splinters and flakes. My right hand holds my legs, touches the coarse hair. I'm trying to become smaller until I disappear entirely. I look at the thin gap, the few inches of space between the bed and the wall, imagining my body slipping down, disappearing completely from view until they – the doctors, the nurses, the other patients – can't see me, can't find me.

The despair and fear comes in waves. The sobs stick inside my windpipe, are occasionally spat out. I put my hand over my mouth, trying desperately to keep my panic private. My breath slows; my lungs fill again. For a moment, three seconds at the most, I'm calm, but it's an expression of optimism and hope that I can't sustain.

As the hands of the clock turn and whir, my nameless, faceless Suicide Preventer is replaced by another. And another. They all look the same. Worried middle-aged women, anxiety stitching the wrinkles into the brows. I look an inch to the left of their face, or an inch to the right. I can't bear to look directly at them and see the sadness, pity, confusion, disappointment painted on their faces, sinking their eyes deep in their faces.

They eventually blur and shimmer and morph into one woman, who sits at the end of my bed on the same small plastic chair tucked into a corner, the drawn curtain brushing her arm. I wonder who she is, who loves her, whom she loves, where she goes home to. Whom she'll tell about the woman who cried and spat and tried to obliterate herself.

In her lap, she clutches the clipboard that they've all been clutching, that holds several sheets of white, lined paper that she must fill in constantly, with tiny words in neat, tight handwriting, covering every movement, every twitch, sniff, glance, every act of mine, however small, however seemingly insignificant. She fills it with wave upon wave of black spidery script, her hand rising and falling with my heartbeat. Later, when I'm more present, I'll become conscious of seeming or not seeming mad, but right now I'm so far away that I don't know and don't care how I seem. It feels so unrelated to me.

34

More patients come in to share my cubicle, sometimes for minutes, sometimes for hours. I don't look at them, acknowledge their presence, their faces beige flat circles with no features.

After some hours in the smudge, the weaving blur, I'm told that I'm about to be taken to the cardiac ward for monitoring. I'll be given medication to detox from alcohol while I'm there, offsetting the vomiting, the shaking, the other physical withdrawal symptoms. I want to walk, but they say I must be pushed and I must be lying in the bed. In a haze of barely remembered, barely registered set of coordinated movements, mostly by other people, I'm moved out of the ER, through the chained, cussing, coughing of the men I pass, to another floor.

My wheels come to a rest and I'm parked in the bay closest to the corridor, artificial yellow light flooding in from two sides: from the streets through the window and from the corridor just to my side. Almost immediately, a slight man with sandy hair comes into view, tossing a small rubber ball against the squeaky floors over and over again.

Bounce, slap, bounce, slap, bounce, slap bounce, slap slap, bounce bounce.

He strides up and down the corridor, past the window facing into the corridor, peers in, the ball a distraction while he hunts out information. I avoid his eyes and draw the curtains.

The current Suicide Preventer is installed at the end

35

of my bed. I look at her, seeking solidarity against Rubber Ball Guy who is already testing my broken mind and patience. She looks my way, not quite meeting my eyes. I stare harder. She doesn't respond, doesn't acknowledge the noise that is repeating and sinking inside my brain, burrowing down.

Slap, slap, bounce, bounce bounce slap.

I move my hands to my head as it repeats and repeats and repeats, echoes in my ears. She studies my reaction, writes, pauses, watches, writes some more. I have my first flash of panic about what she's writing, recording. What if she doesn't get that my enraged look is about how really fucking irritating Rubber Ball Guy is? What if she doesn't see and hear it like I do? And just thinks that I'm, well, nuts? Because I am, right? In here, to her, right now, I'm mad. The gown, the band around my wrist, the file tucked in the end of the bed, they all tell her the same basic, conclusive story: I'm mad. Not to be trusted. Not with myself, not with anyone.

And suddenly I know what my job is. I have to do everything in my power not to seem mad. My face slips into a mask, hardens and I stare at the wall over her shoulder impassively, without evident emotion.

I fall asleep and when I wake up it's three a.m. on the ward. My bed is at the exact point that darkness from the sky and light from the corridor collide, but it's not this that wakes me up. It's the noise coming from the bed next to mine, which has had the curtains drawn around it since I've arrived. All I've seen is scuffling feet;

all I've heard is whispered conversations. But right now, all I hear is:

Beep, beep-beep, beep, beep, beep-beep, beep, beep-beep, beep.

I sit up, now fully awake, irritated. 'Ugh, that noise,' I say to the new Suicide Preventer, a different one to the one who was at the foot of my bed when I went to sleep.

'Noise?' she asks.

I nod. 'Can you hear it?' My hand is to my ear, straining.

She frowns, asks in broken English, 'You hear something?'

I nod again. 'Yes! Do you hear it?'

'Voices?' she asks.

The woman in the cubicle had been talking to the nurse. 'Well, yes, sometimes, but not right n . . .' I start to say, stopping as she immediately starts to write, mouthing quietly to the rhythm of her hand movements.

I settle back into my pillow and then realise what she thinks I just said. 'Hang on! No!' I spring up. 'Not voices!'

'You hear voices,' she says.

'No, no, I don't hear voices! I mean the beeping of the machine, and the voices as they talk.' This is not helping. 'But I don't hear voices that aren't there!'

She looks at me quizzically.

'Please!' I say, trying not to scream. 'Please, if you've written "hears voices" can you please cross it out? I definitely don't hear voices. Not like that.'

She makes a motion to scratch something out but no ink leaves her pen and marks the paper. I ask once more, the exact same question, and she now holds the pen completely still. Tears fill my eyes in panic. I'm making it worse. Every word and movement. I need to stop. I lie back, squeeze my eyes shut and try to breathe through the panic clogging my throat up. I turn on my side away from her, resisting the urge to argue more, to explain more, aware that the situation could possibly get even worse than it currently is.

The next morning, after breakfast, the Suicide Preventer takes me to the shower. I'm given a thin towel and soap. I shuffle to the shower in my hospital gown and socks. We walk inside the shower room. It's a bleak beige room, with dirty tiles and a shower that drips mournfully. I take off my gown and socks, fold them up and place them on the plastic seat by the door. I try to shield my body from her eyes, turn to face the wall and cover my breasts with one hand and turn the tap on with the other. The water that spits out is cold, flecks my body wet as I try to get myself clean.

The Suicide Preventer tuts. I turn my head over my shoulder. 'Why would you do this?' she says. I frown. 'You have a beautiful body, you do. So why would you do this?'

A few hours later, my twenty-four-hour cardiac observation is complete and I'm waiting to be taken to the psychiatric ward upstairs.

'When will I be leaving?' I ask the nurse.

She frowns, looks at my chart. 'Oh, well, it's pretty much always full,' she says. 'It could be several days'.

My stomach falls. 'What?' I say. 'That's not possible. They said that I can't start my psychiatric observation until I'm on the ward – if it's days and days I could be in here weeks.'

She shrugs and walks away.

On the third day, I demand to see the hospital's psychiatrist, a kindly old man with crumpled skin and thick glasses. There's very little he can do, he says. They can't move me up until someone else is ready to leave and they have no clue when that will be. I cry, sobs from my gut and he steps forwards, seemingly moved somewhat. 'We could try to get another hospital to take you. If they have another bed. And depending on your insurance.'

I grasp onto the thin sliver of light. 'Yes, oh, please. What do I need to do?'

The psychiatric team find me a bed at a hospital uptown, but it's one that needs my insurance company to approve my treatment before admission. I call my insurance company. A robot on the phone tells me that they have seventy-two hours to process the request. I splutter. 'Seventy-two hours? No, no, please. You have to sort it faster. I'm stuck in hospital. I'm trapped – please help me.'

They promise to call back. There is no call. The doctors stay away from my bedside. On Wednesday, four days after that terrible morning in the ER, an orderly arrives by my bed. My heart leaps. I must be being taken upstairs.

'Sorry, miss,' he says. 'We're just moving you to another ward.'

I'm taken to a half-empty ward, full of quiet and the light from a perfect blue moonlit sky. My bed is tucked by the farthest window. I spent hours dreaming of the Empire State Building. She was why I'd moved here. The promise, the hope, the opportunity and bottled, captured joy she held. With her reflected in my eyes, I felt like everything, all of it, was possible. But not right now. Right now, she looks like despair, like betrayal. Like sadness and sorrow. How could she lie to me like this? I sleep in her shadow, dreaming of climbing up her elegance, sitting astride the top, squatting over her, making her submit to my pain.

CHAPTER 5

Finally, I'm told it's happening, definitely. That my bed is ready and that an ambulance will be here to transport me. I wake up at dawn, excited as though it's 25th December.

I eat breakfast, take a shower under supervision and then sit on the bed, waiting for my morning transfer. I'm not allowed to wear my own clothes, so I'm in a fresh backless patterned hospital gown and socks.

I've pinned the beehive that has been resting in the bedside unit drawer to my head. Bun piece, as high and erect as possible, then a grey sock folded over to cover it, then two pieces of matted clip-in hair, then my own hair, pinned tight, sprayed stock-still with lacquer. My scalp winces and pulsates under the tug and the pull and the push it hasn't felt now for almost a week. It is the longest time I've had my hair down, unpinned, worn 'naturally', in several months. I won't even go to the bodega on the corner of my block without it normally, but quite honestly, the fact that I don't look like 'myself', have my head armour, has been the least of my worries. And I've found salvation and a safety of sorts in hiding, incognito without my trademark look. I don't want anyone to know who I am and what I'm doing there.

I know how ridiculous I must look, building it straight up, at a ninety-degree angle, while the other patients and their friends and families look on bemused, but it's the only way I can cling on to the tiny bit of me I still know, or at least recognise. And I need it, in this moment, more than ever.

I need to start rebuilding myself, even if just the exterior. It's time to paint my face, over features which have been left blank. I wipe foundation over my skin, becoming an empty page, erasing before I can colour myself into being again. I take the jet-black liquid eyeliner from the inner corners of my eye across and flick up at the sides. Blackest black mascara on each individual lash. Deep red lipstick stains my mouth into a violent permanent smile.

I pack the few items of clothes a friend has snatched for me from my apartment. My wardrobe is normally a carefully cultivated mishmash of second-hand dresses, shirts, skirts, T-shirts. Taken as separate pieces they look like the wardrobe of a deranged woman, but put together, it's something approaching a look. A look that I could hide – exist safely – within. Grabbed at random, however, none of it worked. But it's all I have with me to take to the next hospital: my wardrobe for the psych ward. My pink A-line dress; white shirt; a knee-skimming black dress that sticks to me in the bits that matter and those that don't; a dogtooth mini skirt; an oversized T-shirt for my friend's punk band; thick white tights; off-colour ankle socks; black tights with a ladder by the gusset; vintage lace-up brogues; a striped blue, white and red shirt with a dagger collar; navy blue cropped trousers; a thick yellow mini skirt.

I place my clothes, along with my make-up, a hairbrush and toiletries – moisturiser, hairspray, deodorant – and my laptop neatly in the big transparent plastic bag I've been allocated. The bags that you're given when you leave or join an institution – a care home, a prison, a hospital. The sign that your belongings are, were, never really yours. They belong not just to whoever had given them to you, but to the world. The people who now have every right to see your knickers and your socks and your lipstick on display.

I wait. And wait. Visitors to surrounding beds come and go. The food trolley goes past en route to other beds. 'None for me,' I remind the porter with a smile, 'I'm going to be out of here any minute!' On the hour, every hour, I walk to the nurses' station, still smiling while anxiously asking for an update. 'It's on its way,' they say, on the hour, every hour. As each hour passes, I become more and more anxious. I can't spend another night here in this ward, simply waiting.

It has taken several tear-fuelled conversations to my insurance company and the hospital administration team to sort the bed in the psych ward out for me. If it's lost,

I'll be sent to the back of the queue. I feel beyond desperate just thinking about it.

I sit, stand, pace; I ask again. I don't want to go to the bathroom in case they come and leave without me. The sun sinks a little lower. My bladder remains full. My fingers leave marks in the sides of the chair.

Eventually, several hours later, the paramedics appear: my rescuers. A middle-aged man and a young woman, swinging her high, tight ponytail, chewing gum. 'We've had the worst day,' they say to no one in particular as they pass the nurses' station to collect me. They leave the gurney they were pushing in the corridor and come to the side of my bed.

'Right,' they say. 'Time to get you on there.'

'No thanks!' I chirp, standing bolt-straight to attention as they invite me to get on the stretcher.

The female paramedic shakes her head. It's not a request. 'You have to,' the man then chips in. 'And we have to strap you in. It's procedure.'

I look at the body-shaped stretcher, take a moment to steady myself. The thought of being strapped down, unable to move, takes the breath straight out of my body. They wait. Eventually, I climb up, covering my backside, as they ask me to cross my arms over my body, pull first a sheet then a blanket over me and strap me definitely not in, but down – tight, with black belts pulled across my body. They start to wheel me out and this is the exact moment the trembling starts at my ankles: an immediate, physical manifestation of the panic blossoming, opening wide, in my chest. I can't move. I can't breathe. *Help me. Please. God.* I don't know who I'm looking at, for, but not for the first time that week, I look up. Up through the ceiling tiles, the electrical cables, the concrete, the tiles, the clouds, into the stratosphere, the sky beyond the sky we cannot see, no matter how hard we try.

As they continue wheeling me through the corridors to the elevators, the eyes of other patients and their family members fall on me, before bouncing swiftly away. Everyone can see the madness. The shame. They don't want to be touched by it. There aren't many other reasons to be tied down. I smile widely, red filling my cheeks. The skin in the corners of my mouth cracks, ever so slightly. My smile freezes still. They push me into the lift, talking over me; she casually texts; they laugh. As we get to the exit, my heart leaps. Through the doors, I can see the sunshine, the sky, the people hurrying, the cars speeding: New York, alive right there, just feet away.

I haven't been outside, on concrete, felt the wind, tasted New York's dirty air on my tongue, in almost a week. As the gurney pushes the external doors open with a bang of metal on metal, the air flies in and I instinctively open my mouth, gulping it down. If my hands had been free, I'd have been clutching at it, greedy with need. In the following seven or eight seconds it takes them to push me from the hospital exit to the ambulance doors, the wall of sun, wind, noise, clamour, chatter hits me square in the chest. Sirens collide with horns, meet screeching tires, melded with screams.

The paramedics continue to chat cheerily over my head, seemingly immune to the miracle happening all around us. Then they push me into the ambulance and slam the doors shut, shutting off my New York air supply. The ride uptown can't take more than thirty minutes, but each one of them stretches out like an elastic hour. Not being able to move when you feel panicked is terrifying. Every bit of your body wants to thrash, pull against the ties and make a run for it. But you don't. You lie very still, not moving a muscle, trying to forget you have muscles, a body under the belts, blanket, sheet. You breathe in and out, close your eyes, head on chest. The sounds rage outside but inside the only noise is the tap-tap-tap of the young ambulance tech texting on her phone. When we pull up to a stop and I open my eyes, she has a small smile playing on her face. She looks so free. In that moment, I hate her.

They wheel me into the hospital, up in the elevator, and then we're buzzed in from behind locked double doors. As they push me past the room I'll come to learn is for breakfast, lunch, dinner, supper, chair yoga, music therapy, group therapy, a row of heads turn around, their eyes landing on the new arrival. I keep looking straight ahead.

CHAPTER 6

My life began a long way from New York, in the village of Inkersall, just north of the Derbyshire town of Chesterfield. It was 1975 when my mum and dad first collided. My mum, running from her short life; my dad static, propping up the bar of the rough pub they met in. She was fifteen and living in a house teetering on a fault line. Perhaps the path to each other had already been forged, was simply waiting to be walked.

Her mother, my grandmother, loved to go out dancing and my grandfather loved to drink. He would be dead at fifty-six, their marriage burning and boiling up until the moment he died of a heart attack. Nana fingered the single earring, orphaned decades earlier by a blow to the head outside the working men's club. She told the story of the night he broke her nose, blood spraying long and high up the wall of their neat front room. This was the world in which my mum lived, learned who she was and what she wanted.

Their love crackled bright and quick after a chance meeting in the pub and a wedding was quickly arranged for the day after her sixteenth birthday. My grandad, horrified and furious, made Mum an offer: a horse in exchange for her calling off the wedding. She loved riding more than pretty much anything; anything, it would seem, except my dad. The offer was swiftly rejected, the source of much claimed regret in decades to come.

In another quick act of perhaps easy-seeming rebellion, my brother was in her belly almost as quickly as they became hitched, entering the world a month before her seventeenth birthday. I joined them one year and 364 days later.

Much is disputed, but what isn't is that their marriage was a disaster. He was jealous. He wouldn't work. Their fights turned physical but only after Grandad died. When there were no other men around to protect Mum's face, her body. Before long she was painted with bruises and waiting for the latest broken bone to fuse back together. There was a story she shared of the time she was pregnant, punched to the floor and kicked in her swollen belly. Another, of the Christmas she couldn't see the turkey across the table; both eyes blackened and swollen completely shut, my newly widowed Nana closed-mouthed beside her, warned not to make it worse, because worse it could be. Still another, of the time he outlined, graphically, what would happen if she left him (as she eventually did), how he'd set fire to the house with us all inside.

Mum wasn't his only target. He picked my brother off the ground by both ears and threw him against the wall. He punched me into the fireplace and sat on Mum as she screamed on the settee and I screamed for her in the ashes. That was the one, she says, that prompted her, finally, to take us and leave.

We escaped to Nana's and he didn't, in fact, set fire to us. The memories in the decade that follow are hazy, incomplete. There was, very quickly, a new, younger woman. Blonde with 'CUT' and dotted lines tattooed across both wrists, she was from one of our town's toughest families. He drove a three-wheeled Reliant Robin, and the rare times we would visit him, we'd sit in the back, over the wheels, heads bouncing into the low ceiling.

They married quickly too, his reception in the working men's club ending with linked arms and 'You'll Never Walk Alone'.

The second White Family lived just six miles away, yet they only featured in snatches of my early life. There was a campsite holiday, our bags hastily packed after Dad knocked on the door unexpectedly after another extended absence. Upon arrival, my brother and I were sent to a small pouch in the back of the big family tent, which backed into a hedge. The rest of them slept together in the main section. At night, we sat with them in the communal area, drank Scrumpy out of brown bottles and listened to horror stories about murderers and ghosts and psychopaths before we skipped quickly back beneath the hedgerow. On the second night, while we were sleeping, the spending money Mum had given us to share for the week disappeared.

That holiday was a one-off, and for the most part, when it came to my dad it was waiting and wondering: where was he? When would we next see him? There was one afternoon in their house when we watched him kick his Alsatian dog with the steel toe of his boot. There were the days we spent cleaning his house – every room, every floor, every inch – exhausted by the time we were dropped home. They weren't the memories you would cradle and keep safe.

I recall sitting on top of the sofa, my head stuck through the blinds, waiting, as he never arrived to take me to see Santa at the Co-op as promised. The hours ticked by. One of his – so I suppose by extension our – close relatives was getting married. It was my eleventh birthday. I remember turning up at the door of the fancy hotel in town, and being told that we couldn't come in. That there had been a mistake. That we were not allowed into the 'day do'. That there was no seat for us, no food for us. I tried to look around the big immovable man in the doorway, tried to see Dad so that he could come and save us. But I remember not being able to find him and us being sent away, back out into the street and being told to wait there for a few hours, until we were allowed in.

I was wearing a new dress, my perm tight and rigid. The temperature dropped as the sun dipped and my new, already much-loved Tammy Girl frock offered little warmth. As we sat on a bench by the roundabout in the shadow of the hotel, the sky turned black and I started to cry. My defiantly dry-faced brother – who was already my eternal protector at just thirteen – comforted me. After more time passed and we still weren't allowed inside, I remember walking to a phone box and reversing the charges to ring Mum and that Dad later claimed it had been a 'mix-up'. My cheeks burned at the thought of him sitting inside – scraping his plate clean, while his children were exiled – in the belief that he didn't really want us, never had.

Until then, I'd always fantasised about being a daddy's girl. It was a dream that I tangled in between my fingers and tried to make real in my fists. It had first bloomed in my brain at around six or seven years old: the age I first understood that my life and that of kids around me didn't line up. Through the smudged lenses of my thick NHS glasses, I hungrily watched my friends with their fathers, devoured their casual interactions. The light way they laughed, how their fingers entwined easily, the gentle care of a jacket being zipped all the way up to the chin. It always amazed me to see the dads waiting nervously as we clambered off the bus from the school trip or when they poked their heads gingerly around the door as we wrapped up at Brownies. It all just served to make me ask: I had a dad out there, so why wasn't I good enough to be his girl?

But now, as disappointments piled up and my desperation to be a daughter waned, I resigned myself to being without a dad. Just as well: contact petered out altogether before I began secondary school. His position appeared to be that we knew where he was if we wanted to see him. We did, and I for one didn't in the face of his ambivalence. Until I turned seventeen. Then I became suffocated by the need to find out who this man was. To find out who *I* really was. It was teatime on Boxing Day when I knocked on his door.

'Hello, duck,' he said, seemingly only moderately surprised, vaguely pleased to see me. I went in, had a cup of tea, we made polite conversation, I left. Hopes of a restorative process, leading to a real father–daughter relationship proved, to me, overly optimistic, impossible. In the preceding years I'd watched *Surprise Surprise* avidly, imagining *our* reunion: the tears, the joy, the feeling of coming home. But looking into his eyes – so much like mine – I felt no rush of love, no sense that I was inextricably his. I was sure he felt the same. We kept up sporadic visits nonetheless. His wife would take us walking through graveyards at midnight, on the hunt for ghosts. Other than that, we sat in uncomfortable silence in front of the TV as horse racing and the bloated voices of those who narrated it roared out.

It finally ended not unlike it began. I was nineteen and leaving for a summer abroad. It was also my birthday. He was coming round to 'say goodbye' after he'd turned me away from his door earlier in the day, when I'd arrived unexpectedly with a Father's Day gift. 'I'll be there by seven p.m.,' he promised, buying time, time he'd pocket, never intending to use.

I sat by the window and waited, each set of passing

headlights a fresh disappointment. As I started to cry, I remembered the almost identical scene when I'd been waiting to see Santa. When I'd sat and waited, refused to come out of the window. When I'd allowed myself to be strung up in misery. He hadn't come then, and he wasn't going to come now. He would never come, never realise his responsibilities. At four a.m., I closed the blinds and wiped my face. As I walked up the stairs I thought: the question really was not where was he but *who* was he? I didn't know him. He wasn't a dad. At least, he wasn't my dad.

Some five or so years later, a brief rapprochement. My phone rang. It was my brother, telling me that Dad was in hospital. His wife had recently died and he'd driven out into the dark countryside lanes and had an accident. He was in intensive care and we were advised to see him while there was time. I took the train and arrived at his bedside, thick, tied tubes lodged in his throat, mouth, machines beep-beeping, pulsating. I felt like a charlatan at his bedside.

Against the odds, he survived; he recovered. Once he did, I recall him promising to be there, to be present, saying how much he missed us, how much he missed me. I felt nothing then, and nothing again when, once again, he disappeared from my life – leaving me with no consoling memory of a goodbye.

CHAPTER 7

Into this gap, the father-shaped hole in my life, walked other men, almost immediately. I never had the chance to hope they would be better men, better fathers than mine had been – it was clear from the start that some were, in fact, much worse. The first that was worse arrived within a year or two of the day we fled Dad.

There was a morning. A morning when I looked at him from where I sat curled up on the sofa. This morning, he was solid. Just yellow hair, white skin, hard bone. Just blood. I knew that if I nicked his thumb with a butter knife, red would run into the blond hair that curled around his wrist, making a crunchy matted knot that tasted like metal as you sucked. It lay heavy and thick on my tongue.

He winked now, safe in his security. 'So,' he said. 'We played wrestling last night. Right?' The first bit was for her; the second was for me.

I giggled and bowed my head. 'Yes.'

She nodded as the acrid smoke from the frying pan snaked and settled into the twists and turns of her perm.

We glanced, co-conspirators now. The familiar shiver and nauseous bloom in my tummy. I laid my arm across to stop it spreading and gripped my second rib, holding myself in place.

Her make-up was smeared and her smell sour, but last night she stood in thick choking clouds of Elnett and perfume. Smoothing down her leather skirt and tilting her head, she'd put the finishing touches to the woman in the small mirror perched on the windowsill over the sink. I could tell she was pleased with what, who she saw. I practised arching my back and raising my cheekbones skyward: first one and then the other.

There was a night. A night that she moved down the hall, carried away on her familiar sweet smell. I clutched at her with sticky fingertips as she glanced my way, irritated by the tiny person she recognised but didn't see.

'What?'

Panic swelled my tongue dormant. 'It'll hap-p-pen,' I managed to stutter, an increasingly frequent occurrence by then, soon to be joined by wetting the bed. 'If you . . . go.'

Her heels hit the uneven steps down the front path as she went. I watched her grow smaller in the frosted glass, until she disappeared entirely. Then there was just me and him under the darkening sky.

I was in my white pyjamas on the orange and brown sofa. My eyes began to fall and close. 'Stay awake,' he urged, prodding my arm. 'You can't go to sleep!' The carriage clock on the mantelpiece said I should be asleep, that I shouldn't be here. I pulled at the loops of loose threads on the cushion as things I didn't understand danced across the TV screen.

'But I'm tired,' I said.

'Stay. Awake.' He stared.

I imagined what I always do when this happens: that matchsticks, half the size of those in my nana's kitchen drawer, are jammed between my eyelids, propping them open. I played it on repeat: *matchsticks, matchsticks, your eyes are open; you're awake. Matchsticks, matchsticks, your eyes are open; you're awake.*

I started to pray. Though I don't understand Him, I'm pretty sure I believed in Him, that God was there. Let me go to bed; I'd do anything, please let me. Eventually He heard because he said: 'You can go up to bed now.'

I climbed the stairs, grateful, scared, hoping that tonight I could just sleep and wake up in the daylight, safe. As my eyes fluttered in my head, the fractured second floorboard let out a hesitant *creeaaakk*. It aborted, drew breath. As he advanced it slowly exhaled a low *moannnnnnn*. The room was black and the thin pink blanket covered my crown, but I could still see him. He was creeping on the raw ends of his toes towards the next door on the left. Propelled by the force that held him by the bare waist, a puppet with shaking joints and a frozen smile, lurching along.

He inched into the light, the shadow on his back

falling, draped behind. The crack beneath the door was still white. I breathed in, sharp, in the second before he seeped through. The edges of the pink blanket were tugged, tugged, tugged as my knuckles turned grey. The fog curled around my ankles, inched up my calves, cupped my knees and coiled the white skin of my thighs as he bargained and pleaded and I was pared, peeled and torn.

'I'll buy you chocolates,' he said, as I folded my lips around him. He never did.

Later, I told someone who told someone else, about the nights my skin was pulled back. There was an afternoon. He'd taken an overdose, was retching, spitting, vomiting, screaming in our toilet. He was crying, begging. His pleas sounded so much like mine. But mine were silent, stored in my belly, and I despised him for his weakness.

'You fucked your "dad",' they said to me at school when my mother's boyfriend's name, our address, my age, ended up in the paper. I found it hard to disagree. The stain seeped inside me, thickened my blood, turned my bones to charcoal. It was part of me now. I'd never be free. He was me and I was him.

When the first men I wanted laid their fingers on me, it was his touch that I felt, his face that I saw. I'd always be his. His thumbs would circle my throat until it fell still.

CHAPTER 8

Peace reigned in our house briefly. We sat in our trauma, the tranquillity licking at our wounds. Time passed.

And then he arrived. The man who would set us off running for a second time. His hands were rage-stacked ships, fully rigged with sovereign rings that shone as they swept and sank. Not at first though. At first, his hands were warm and soft, waiting, welcoming.

I was balanced on his knee, swaying high off the ground. He was reading me a story, his voice emerging from beneath his chest bones. His fingers gently turned the sticky pages that flinched in the sunlight that tricked its way through the net curtains. The front room was full of giggles and dancing dust as I wriggled and looked up at this new man.

I would come to learn that he was the strongest and meanest of men. You learned these things when a man strangled your mum; when a man punched you in the face that was still smaller than his fist.

Before that though was the beginning. They met in

a bar. Mum offered him a place to stay. Her house. Our home. Her bed. Within weeks, it was his home and we were the ones in need of refuge.

The first fist is nowhere in my memory, no matter how much I dig and turn and sift and sort. But the tenth, the twentieth are there. Sometimes it was a full, closed fist and sometimes an open hand or a tightly clenched back of the hand, knuckles bared and braced. I heard the wind rush through the gap between his thumb and first finger as he brought it down from on high, the whoosh being snuffed out by the crack of hand on skin and bone and the scream that would escape my mouth no matter how tight I locked my throat.

A winter's night. It was Sunday. *No Jacket Required* was playing, the car we were in sped along. Cat's eyes counted down the country lanes to home. There weren't enough, there were never enough, to make the journey long enough. My nerves bobbed and weaved as he and Mum traded clipped conversation, faces lit by the swooping headlights of cars as they passed. I imagined the families, the lives, in those cars that were so unlike ours.

By the time we were walking up the uneven path that led to our front door, one foot taken off-balance as usual by the wonky paving, I sensed a shift. My legs began to shake. 'Frozen pizzas for tea?' half-asked Mum.

'Do we have to? I want something else.' Maybe I said this, I can't remember.

'What the fuck?' He came alive with anger, spit rained down. 'There are fucking kids starving in Africa and you're fucking complaining about what you're having for tea! Get here.' I walked over to his balled fists. My body tensed, waiting for the wind. Instead, 'You can get to bed without any tea, you fucking little bastards.' I ran, giddy with relief, and I lay, as I always did, on my bedroom carpet, ear pressed tightly to the floor as shouts and crashes rose. I collected them in my hands, kept them safe.

A summer's afternoon. It was a Saturday. Last night they'd gone drinking, leaving us with a babysitter. He walked into the front room as I folded myself smaller and smaller into the corner of the settee. 'Were you good?' he said, with a face straight and still.

'Yes,' I said. I was. Wasn't I?

'Were you?' he asked again.

I paused. 'Yes,' I said, unsure.

'You little fucking liar. Get here.'

I walked towards him, tiny steps, but steps all the same. He took a single stride to meet me, his arm touched the sky and came crashing down under my chin, sending my body up into the air. For a second, I was flying. I was free. Then my head, followed by the rest of me, landed in the dining room, next to the silent hi-fi. He stood over me, fists blazing red as I waited for the rest.

A spring morning. It was Sunday. They always got up late, delayed by the rhythmic slap, slap, slap of their damp skin. I was awake, careful not to make noise, fearful of the paper-thin wall between this bedroom and theirs. I wasn't careful enough. A lumbering, long creak

60

extinguished by one heavy foot on the floorboards. I breathed in.

'You wake me up? You wake *me* up? Get dressed and get the fuck downstairs.'

I dressed slowly, but not too slowly. As I stood at the top of the stairs, the vomit stung the back of my throat. I knew what was at the bottom. I swallowed it and walked down.

He beat us in the daylight, under the white open sky. But, unbelievably, there was still worse. What he did in the darkness.

An autumn evening. It was Friday. Mum was working in the pub, he was babysitting. I was woken up by him calling my name. I was in my nightie and barefoot as I walked the handful of steps down the landing. Now it was my turn to creep and crawl.

'Yeah?' I asked, nervously.

'Come in,' he said. I opened the door, peered around and he was naked from head to toe.

I knew instantly that it was wrong, that I needed to get away, fast and far, but I also knew not to run. What would happen if I did. So I didn't. One fear overtook the other and I stood perfectly still.

'Come and sit down,' he said. 'Hold this.' I sat cross-legged on the carpet and held the magazine he'd given me. On the pages were pictures of big-breasted women, also wearing no clothes, brown hair shooting out in big curly mounds from between their thighs. 'Hold it the right way up,' he snapped. I froze, confused, until he took it and turned it so it faced him. Relieved, I held it against my chest. I didn't have to look at the pictures, look into the eyes of the women he was hurting. He was cross-legged across from me, holding his penis in his hand.

He moved his hand back and forwards until it got bigger and harder in his fist. I held the magazine in front of my face so I couldn't see. 'Hold it lower,' he shouted, gasping for breath. 'Lower, now.'

Slap, slap, pound, sigh, slap slap.

I did as I was told, inched it down.

'Lower.'

A little more.

'I said lower.'

It occurred to me too late that he wanted me to see. Needed me to see. Small white wet flecks shot out of the end of him and sprayed all over the room. I looked at the ceiling, the Artex charmed me like a snake into another reality. I escaped into it, climbed into the other dimension, my arms opened wide.

The next morning, he held a bacon sandwich. She hadn't trimmed the fat off. We had bacon scissors, useless for anything else, right there in the drawer, but she didn't take them to the task at hand. Just tossed the white, thick rinds into the spitting, kicking oil. The rinds bobbed now, black and hard and curled, in the shallow pool of shimmering grease. They glistened, strangely beautiful in the sunlight.

The chewy slick was a welcome distraction. From

him, from what happened. 'Pass the red sauce,' he said. I picked up the ketchup and reached out my fist. The only part of me still whole. Those fingers brushed bone as I met his eyes and smiled.

I can't remember if he instructed me not to tell, but he didn't need to. I felt ashamed, complicit, smeared with him and knew that I couldn't tell anyone about that night ever.

One day I cried at school, the shame and disgust falling out of me. I told the teacher I was crying because of what happened to me before, when I actually wanted to tell her that I was crying because of what was happening to me now. But I couldn't; I didn't. It was my fault.

Why would both of them do this to me unless I'd welcomed it, wanted it? Why couldn't I see what I must be putting out into the world of men? It was my fault; I just had to take it.

But crying at school was definitely a slip. They called my mum and we were referred to family therapy. We sat in a room separated from another room with glass that I couldn't see through. There were people watching us through the glass.

I looked at the glass, the mirror, saw myself looking back and wondered what they saw, the invisible ones. What did they see when they looked at me? The things that I was trying to hide? The very worst of me?

The woman asked why I was afraid; who and what I was afraid of. He sat two seats away.

'You're safe now,' she said. 'You know that he wouldn't ever do anything like that.'

I nodded, nodded, nodded, resisted the urge to shake my head and scream until my voice bounced off the ceiling and down into his throat, cutting off his air. Instead, I sat mute. The shame, the sickness curdled in my stomach and ran down into my thighs and feet, leaving me still as a statue.

I was so alone in my secrets. And so lost. I no longer existed in the world. I was away, away, away, where the birds flew and flocked.

One morning, after I'd escaped the terror of home, I turned up at the door of the local church. Drawn by the singing, the happiness, the open door. I woke up early every Sunday after – the day they would sleep in until lunchtime – got dressed into any half-decent clean clothes, scrubbed my face bright and then turned up at the door again. It was the only place I felt safe, felt beyond their touch. I looked up, told Him it all. It was the only roof that I ever stood under and spoke the truth; where I didn't feel like I was already dead.

When we did eventually leave him, it was remarkable how unremarkable it was. There had been far worse times. The time he'd discovered Mum drinking a bottle of wine in the middle of the day, dragged her upstairs by the hair, sat on her chest and, knees pinning her arms, took aim and punched until her nose shattered and her fingers snapped and blood sprayed and splattered. The time the knuckles on the back of his right hand had sent me and my brother up into the air in tandem, after my fingers had caught in the kitchen window as we played.

This morning, it began with a crash, a bang and then silence that hung heavier than the thuds that fell in between. Through the wall, I heard the drawers of the dressing table being pulled out. They bounced off the carpet, their contents danced in the air. Angry muffled words flew with them; the quieter responses belonged to her. I sat in my bedroom, hiding in a place where there was no hiding, but at least I wasn't in the thick of the war. More words, spat. The front door slammed, his heavy foot unsettling the second paving slab that led to the gate that led to the street that led to his car, in which he drove away, tyres screaming.

Immediately, something was different. Mum, wide-eyed, whirled around the living room. The one-sided fight had been about the absence of socks in his under-wear drawer. And at the front door, a balled hand and a promise: 'If there aren't any socks in that drawer by the time I get home, you'll be getting some fist.'

We knew that there was nothing my mum could do in the next eight hours to avoid getting some fist, to save the bones in her face. But what Mum said next caught me off-guard.

'Put some stuff in a bag – we're going,' she said. We stood still, didn't move. 'I said get a bag, put some stuff in – we're leaving!' she shrieked, pulling us upstairs. I dug out my favourite bag – a tote bag from the Brownies featuring a smiling girl outside a country cottage, roses around the door.

We left the house – me, Mum, my brother and sister. I still couldn't believe we were really going. What I did believe, though, was that he was going to kill us. He would come back, find us trying to leave and first he would kill Mum and then he would kill us. I saw our bodies, piled on top of each other, our tongues bursting out of our non-moving mouths. I stroked the little girl's face, her features smooth and unchanging under my fingertips. The roses stayed pinned.

We walked out of the door, four more pairs of feet hitting the uneven paving slab as one by one we marched in order. We walked down the street, round the green, past the shops and arrived at the bus stop. We waited for the bus to come bumping, humping down the hill, while in my mind I saw his car come around the corner, coming for us. The bus stop was exposed on both sides, including the left-hand side his car would appear from, catching us in his headlights. I tried to look for an escape route, but could see only capture.

I thought of our dog, who had been on the end of his boot a hundred times or more. She would hide under my bed, curled into the tiniest ball as he hunted her, before making a desperate bid for freedom along the radiator, his outstretched fingers and ends of his feet straining for the edges of her fur. He always caught her, her howls alerting us to the fact that he had, that he'd found her ribs, was enjoying the moment of pleasure from feeling his steel toe pin her to the hot metal. And now, we'd left her at home to run. And if he couldn't kill us, he would kill her.

But we had nowhere to go and no one to save us — he knew my nana, who lived just a few streets away, and my mum's few remaining friends who also lived in our village. Mum had no money of her own. And so, we pitched up in the place that those with no hope go: the Citizens Advice Bureau. We sat first behind a desk facing a harried woman who listened to the basics of Mum's story, our story, while we piled silently onto one seat. We were then spoken to in a private room. I heard Mum. 'He's going to hit me tonight . . . He said I'd get some fist . . . He strangled me on the settee after I said I didn't want his baby.'

The lady softened, began to call around, searched for a safe place, a refuge. There weren't many places that could take three kids, I learned very quickly. She called, her voice dropped, the phone went down. She called, her voice dropped, the phone went down. The fear in my belly grew. But then – good news. There was a refuge that could take us – the last one with any room in the country. I'd never been out of our town. We were given money for the train we couldn't afford, warned to go straight to the station without telling anyone. We were still in danger. This is when most women die.

We arrived safely at the refuge, walked up tall steps, knocked on an imposing door and, once the person on the other side had established who we were, we were let inside the house. The refuge was full of women and children who looked just like us – our mirror image, over and over: small, brittle and terrified. Women who needed to be invisible but were alert for the fight they weren't yet sure they didn't need to have. The fear was hot, thickened the air. There was a panic button linked through to the local police station. I wondered how many minutes, how many seconds, the door would hold under a boot.

The other children had knotty hair, balled fists, dirty knuckles and wild, suspicious eyes. The women clutched mugs of tea and spoke in small, sore sentences. It was the first time I'd heard accents other than ours being spoken and the sound of their singing belied the brutality of their song. One had left when her husband finally stabbed her after years of beatings. She'd run before, but he'd found them. He would find them again, she said. He always found them. Her girls twirled around her words, knotted hair dancing. She would go home to him, sorrys accepted, just days later. He'd found them.

We had our own bedroom but shared a bathroom, a kitchen, a living room. There were rules: everyone did chores and contributed to the running of the house. We weren't to tell anyone the address of the house, or that the house was a refuge. Breaking that rule would be when the men came. At that point, our only protection would be the female workers in the refuge.

On the second day that we lived in the house that didn't officially exist, I found it: a book on UFOs and alien abductions, tucked in the back of the cupboard under the telly, giving voice to those taken in the dead of night. They all spoke the same language, a language that I recognised: of bright lights, cold metal and paralysing fear. I read it, their stories, over and over, carrying it everywhere, always, tucked under my arm as I moved from room to room. At night, I lay with it beneath me, waiting for the men to come as darkness fell and the moon looked away.

During the daytime, I now went to a nearby school, where everyone spoke words I couldn't decipher, who looked even more alien: they ran through the playground so free and *carefree*. So absent of pain. I stood on the edges of the playground silently, clutching my book. My nights were spent waiting to be taken. When I slept, I'd dream that they were violating and breaking my body under their yellow glare. Long, lumpy fingers jabbed at my skin, pushed inside into my bones, pulled them out to stare at and snap.

I heard that he was looking for us. He turned up at Nana's house. He cried. *Cried.* I tried to imagine him crying, my face scrunching in concentration. I saw him sitting in my nana's front room, on her green two-seater sofa. On his face were cut-out tears on white paper, coloured in blue felt-tip, stuck on with Sellotape folded into small squares.

Then one day, several weeks later, just like that, we were going home. He'd gone, apparently. We'd be 'safe'. But he knew where we lived; he had keys. I didn't feel safe.

The first day we got back, the neighbour next door shouted up from the path by her back door.

'We would hear you all screaming,' she said, then paused. 'We thought about calling the police. But we didn't want to interfere.'

One unremarkable day, years later, when he was long gone, she found it: the one place I'd committed the truth to record – my diary. I wrote every day, confessing, sharing all of the things that would no longer fit in my head, in my body, which was overwhelmed, unwilling. I told it everything.

She called me downstairs. She'd been drinking. I'd been sloppy in hiding it. I'd described the nights, the magazine, the slap, slap and the white specks. She asked me, is it true? I told her yes, it's true.

The next day, I came home from school and she was hoovering the front room. When I walked in, she turned it off with her foot. She asked if I wanted to go to the police about what we'd talked about the night before, or just forget about it. I said I just wanted to forget about it.

She nodded, kicked the hoover and it roared into life once more. We never spoke of it again.

CHAPTER 9

I knew from a very young age that we were poor. Not just struggling, or skint, but poor. A knowledge that instilled fear, insecurity. Hope, optimism was not a familiar taste. I was anxious, constantly. There were the days not answering the door, the phone. The muttered comments at school from parents and their kids.

'Scrubber,' said my best friend. 'Their house is disgusting.'

A house her mum and dad didn't want her to come to. They laughed at our yellow teeth, our dirty clothes; they knew, somehow, that we only had one bath a week.

There was the sometimes-empty pantry and fridge. The food that we did have didn't always stretch. The hunger. The fresh milk in the door that was to last through tens of cups of tea, that we absolutely weren't to drink on its own. I sipped it out of the bottle after dark, in the light of the fridge, and then replaced it with water, the level monitored and marked.

But still we needed, wanted stuff. And stuff cost money. Thankfully, there were always solutions for families like

71

ours. Solutions that cost money, in a way that it didn't for those more fortunate.

The man from Shopacheck came by every Friday night, through our front door into the front room. He wore a beige suit, a camel shirt, a fat brown tie, had thick bifocal glasses and a parting kept in place with what he said was pomade but looked like gel. He'd hold his book, the one in which he marked down all the money Mum owed, the smaller amounts she paid back, and a key. The key was for our telly, which had a coin-operated meter on the back (all your entertainment needs! 50p a go!).

Every week, he emptied the slot, the clatter-clatter of coins falling out into the palm of his hand. He placed them inside his deep pockets, alongside a thin pile of notes from Mum's hand. She flirted with him as she handed over the cash, laughed at his jokes, presumably thinking that one week she might need to rely on his previously unseen generous nature. Meanwhile we sat on the sofa, watching this man warily. Another man who looked at Mum like they were eyeing meat swinging on a hook.

We never had quite enough 50ps. The TV was practically all we had for entertainment, so the tick-tick-tock of the timer counting down was particularly taunting. There were very few books in our house, bar tatty thrillers and bodice-rippers. There were no cinema trips, museums, parks, play centres. There was just a bare bedroom, the green outside the house or the patch of carpet in front of the telly.

When there were no 50ps left, and therefore no TV, I fled to the trees, inched up them, hands scraped by the bark, the fear at my back pushing me to climb higher. Branch to branch to branch until I was hidden in the canopy, finding safety under the leaves that tickled my scalp. I looked over the houses that sat snugly side by side up and across the estate and imagined I lived in one of them. I envisioned pulling up a chair at a table in these strangers' home, being one of their children they loved *so* much. They brushed my hair gently, smoothed down stray damp strands each time the comb was pulled through. Swallowed me up in a smothering hug, the soft perfume of my non-mother filling my throat as my non-father smiled at us across the warm room.

When I hid in the leaves, I was hiding not just from the real but from the imagined. And I couldn't honestly tell the difference between the two. There was a raised bump – or was it a lump? – in the middle of my head, just on the back to the right. I was twelve when I first noticed it – why hadn't I before? I examined it constantly, fingers probing. It was hard yet soft in places, rising up out of my skull. A mess, a mass of bone, flesh and blood, barely covered by my thin hair: a brain tumour, I was sure of it.

I read the big grey *Reader's Digest Medical Book* with

one hand and rubbed my probable tumour with the other. I checked the symptoms off one by one:

Headache (yes. Pretty sure)
Nausea/vomiting (I had felt sick the other day)
Fatigue (I was always tired)
Drowsiness (I was fairly sure I rolled on my
    heels in the dinner queue the other week)
Memory problems (had I?)

I touched it, rubbed it, kneaded it, a hundred times a day. I knew the shape and scale and slope of it. I knew that each morning it had grown just a little bit longer, larger, taller. Life was now split into two time frames: before and after I felt it, noticed its presence. I definitely remembered the former, even if I couldn't feel how relatively carefree my life had been without the worry of impending death weighing heavily on my skull.

Alongside the tumour, I had AIDS. And the question wasn't going to be if I died but when and who I took with me by spreading my sickness. I thought of the dark nights in my bedroom, my mouth around him and I knew that's how you got it, how I'd got it.

I stopped drying my face on the towels in the bathroom and used my sleeve instead. I turned the head of my toothbrush away from the others. I thought of all of us using one toilet seat and added up the likelihood of me infecting everyone else in the family. They'd go out in the world and it would be stuck to them like acid rain. They'd touch the hands of others, it would stick to them and on it would go until I'd killed the world dead.

As I sat on the floor in the front room, the TV blared dire warnings of death punctuated by close shots of gravestones. Sombre-faced middle-aged TV presenters warned us about the modern plague. The thud of gravestones falling echoed around the chamber of my chest. Was now the right time to tell everyone about my sickness? To warn them? But I didn't. I pulled my knees close to my chest and turned into myself. If I could get small enough, if I could become invisible then everyone would be safe.

Eventually part of me broke, it must have done, because I convinced Mum to take me to the doctor. There I sat across from the man who'd tended to my family's health for decades and told him, face burning, that I had AIDS and was going to die and that I'd probably infected my entire family. He looked faintly bewildered, a small smile playing on his lips while the rest of his face remained a mask of composure.

'OK,' he said. 'Let's run through the ways you get it.' He talked about drugs and sharing needles and dangerous sex and gay men and blood blending with blood. I wanted to tell him that I'd had oral sex. That was how and why I knew I had it. But I couldn't. I didn't. How could I? I knew he'd think I was a slut. So I looked down, allowed him to finish, didn't say a word.

Seven years later, I was in my bedroom, the hi-fi was

playing the news. The DJ said something about the world ending; attuned to catastrophe, my ears pricked up. He talked about Nostradamus, who predicted future events, many correctly, how he said the world would end in a nuclear war in the year 2000. It was 1993. Everything stopped. I'd just been given a death sentence; we all had. I found books in the library that told me what to expect, that painted the future for me in black. There would be no plants, no animals, no humans. The earth would be scorched and stripped of everything that made it what it was now. It was all I could think about. I cried for hours, wished that life could have been different. It seemed particularly cruel. I'd be twenty-one. I would finally be free and life would be something other than sadness and pain and then I'd die.

As we drove along in the car and I looked out of the window at the fields we passed, I looked at the cows, imagined their bones burned to dust and then blown away into the air, mixing with all the bone dust of everything and everyone else that had perished when the nuclear bombs landed. I imagined the life I could have had, should have had. It was the first thing I thought of when I woke up every morning, the last thing I thought of when I went to sleep. Everything seemed utterly pointless when death was so close. Every blue sky or toasty summer's day seemed just to exist to demonstrate what we were set to lose.

The six-week holidays were the worst time of all. Six weeks without the distraction of school to occupy my mind; six weeks for my obsessions and anxiety to spiral; when I needed comfort more than ever. But Mum couldn't bear kids under her always moving feet. She was irritated by the very sight of us, around so much, reminding her that we existed.

'I'm going to change my name if you keep using it,' she'd say as we called out 'Mum'. I didn't know much about mothering, or what a typical family looked like, sounded like, felt like, but I knew that a mother should nurture, protect and love their children. I wanted her to hold me, shelter me from the bombs when they fell, take the force of the nuclear blast for me, tell me she loved me as I died.

I don't recall any touching in our house and I grew up desperate to feel skin on mine. To be hugged, swaddled, swept up in an embrace. To be kissed on the head, on the cheek, told how much I am loved. I don't remember there being a single expression of love, either from hands or mouth.

The bubble around me and the world grew. I looked at the other kids around me as if they were aliens – which, to me, they were. They looked like me on the outside only. I couldn't talk to them, relate to them. I spent my days inside, reading anything that had words on it – newspapers, dog-eared thrillers, bodice-rippers, the backs of packets and tins. I watched men in bright tights wrestle each other on TV, swept away by the fantasy world they created.

'Why don't you have any friends and play out like a

normal kid?' Mum asked, at the end of her tether, seeming to be sick of my small, dark presence floating around the house like a ghost. I couldn't explain to her that I felt so apart from all of them. Like I'd been dug up out of the earth, made to look like a child when, really, I was something else. I sat; I stood. I read. I wrote stories that took me away on pirate ships, eye patch strapped on, hat askew, as I led my men and my ship bounced on the rough sea.

But at night, I couldn't hide. I had to go to sleep. And as I lay in the top bunk, my mind raced, filled with images and sounds. I knew they were going to come for me. When everyone else was asleep and I was still awake, they would come. There was no keeping them out. No chains, no locks, no barriers strong enough. I daren't sleep, because that would let them in, but when I couldn't fight it any longer and my mind and body closed down, they were in my dreams. Or were my dreams just memories? They appeared in through the ceiling, walked straight through the bedroom door, came in the windows to my right shoulder. They brought me home to my bed each time but I also knew that there might come a time that they decided not to, when I'd be lost forever.

The nights I didn't dream of being taken, I dreamt about dying, of being killed. I felt the sharp edge of the knife inside my chest, snaking, as it made its way through bone to the fat and the organs below. The knife was pulled and jammed back in over and over. The skin opened, blood rushed in and filled the hole, spilled out of the sides all over my skin. I turned from white to pink to scarlet red, lying in a river of my own blood. I didn't scream or fight or twist and turn. I didn't try to escape. I submitted to the violence, to the pain that poured over me. I knew that I was dying and I was relieved.

My mind was twisted and torn, but really it was my body that I wanted to destroy. First I had to reclaim it. I knew it had been taken from me, stolen by those who had no right, who took it without asking, who took it with balled fists and set jaws and stuffed it, broken and bowed, into the corner. I wanted to reclaim it and then I wanted to destroy it. To light a match and watch it burn. My mind would finally quieten as the flesh blistered and shrank.

Ever since I could remember I'd wanted to make my skin sting, my eyes burn, my insides bleed. I broke rulers, careful to let the end form into a point sharp enough to slice my skin open until, at last, I saw red. Snapped biros between my teeth and scratched at my thighs until they were inflamed; bits of plastic sat inside new rivets. I hit myself in the head and recognised the pain and jolt of my brain banging against my skull momentarily. I pulled at the skin under my eyes and wondered how hard I'd have to pull to tear it off my face entirely.

I had a brown bottle filled to the top with blue capsules. I wasn't sure what they were or why I was taking them. I rolled the lid between my thumb and forefinger and imagined the relief if I took one, two, three, four, five until the bottle was empty. I knew very little but I did know that existing was painful, too painful, already. Every second of my existence was pain. All I wanted was for it to end. I was just twelve years old.

CHAPTER 10

I f it was escape I longed for, there was one sure-fire route to oblivion, well trodden by members of my family, going back generations.

The first time alcohol touched my lips, I wasn't yet as tall as the mantelpiece: the taste delivered by a few slurps out of a can of cheap lager from the Spar, handed to me by my mum.

But it was so much more than how it tasted. Boy, did it make me *feel*. The warm, beautiful, bouncing buzz didn't stay just in my belly – it flowed, flooded down into my thighs, floated to my chest and curled up inside my head. There it sat; it settled, for a moment, cotton wool around my brain, protecting it from the bruises, momentarily filling in the scars. And for that moment, I held my breath and felt something remarkable, something that I struggled to recognise when it began. I was comfortable, standing right there in the world, wearing this skin. A feeling I'd forgotten, if I'd ever in fact had it. Shoulders back, stomach out, spine straight. I felt brilliant and bold. My bones rattled, my body flinched and jerked, as if I'd been plugged into the mains, the dial turned up to ten.

The second time, it was the same hand – my mother's – reaching out, offering more, more, more. Smiling as I shyly accepted. Now I swam around the room bobbing up and down, in and out, swimming, sinking, drowning, surviving. My ideas were bigger, my visions brighter. Colours popped and jumped and kicked and caressed my eyeballs. I wasn't just ready to face the world but straining at the leash. The collar around my neck that kept me quiet, kept me small and scared, was stretching, ready to buckle and break under my new will.

I was in my teens: it was the night Mum fought with another of the men in her life – the man who we, she, had to ask permission from. His particular torment for us was control, not sexual violence.

Can I use the car?

Can I turn the TV on?

Can I turn the TV over?

Can I have a bath?

Can I go out?

Can I speak?

Can I drink the milk?

Can I read the newspaper?

Can I listen to music?

Can I have some money?

Can I have a drink?

Can I love my own children?

Tonight, she snapped and kicked out from under the

suffocation of his control, freeing her head first and then her body. Words were spat and she stormed out of the living room, over the lino in the kitchen and out of the back door, grabbing her purse and me – 'Terri, come on' – as she went.

I jumped up without a second's thought, figuring there'd be punishment but buoyed by the slightest chance that this time she was busting herself, us, out for good.

Once we were down the path and over the green we looked at each other wild-eyed, high on disobedience and the prospect of freedom, however brief. We turned left at the bottom of the road and walked up the winding streets of the estate. We reached the corner shop, halfway up the estate, where she bought the cheapest cider and lager they sold, litre bottles of each; she'd loosened the cap before we'd even left the shop.

She marched quickly, furiously swigging from the bottle while she told me in detail how much she hated him and why. How he controlled her. How he wanted to crush who she was. How insecure and weak he was. How she was so, so sick of staying quiet, being good.

I hated him, too. For all the reasons she said and so many more she didn't. 'You should be seen and not heard,' he'd say and I'd spend days and nights sitting quietly, my thoughts and arguments and resentments screaming around the edges of my mind while a man who couldn't even begin to match me told me why I wasn't worth anything and would always be 'nothing'.

After each swig and swallow and sprayed sentence,

she passed me the plastic bottle. Both hands around its girth, I put it to my lips and sucked, the bottle collapsing in the middle: the liquid fizzed and burned in my too-small throat as I trotted alongside her, struggling to keep up. We walked for what felt like hours; we walked and talked until we'd walked and talked in circles. There was nowhere to go, just around the estate, round and round, where our world began and ended and began again.

The sun had set long ago and the air had turned cold. We had no coats; we were just wearing T-shirts and jeans. The bottles were hollow now, the bottom boasted just an inch of liquid. Home was inevitable; he was inevitable. We crashed from the cascading highs of daring to defy him and started to walk back, slowly and solemnly now. Orange street lights guided our weaving way.

As we walked up the path, I saw the TV still blaring through the living room – he was definitely home and definitely up – and realised quite how drunk I was, though the whole concept was still relatively new to me. Raging, roaring, roll-around-in-a-hedge drunk. My stomach leapt and lurched with the weight and acidity of the booze as we skulked in, heads bowed. He sat waiting, watching the snooker with the volume down low, not speaking, smoking, sucking hard on the cigarette butt clasped tightly between his fingers. His cheeks caved in every time he pulled and I could see every bone in his skull, the way he'd look when he was dead. It was a gift, a power that I'd decided alcohol had given me.

I sat on the carpet, seeing two of every wild, bright swirl that curled under my crossed legs. There were four men taking it in turns to pot balls on two snooker tables on the one TV in front of me. After a few minutes it was eight men potting balls on four snooker tables on two TVs. I lost count of how many should be there, so closed first my left eye and then my right. I needed to focus. Concentrating hard, tongue between my damp lips, the men continued to multiply and duplicate until there was an army of them with blue-tipped sticks and square glasses and tightly tied waistcoats that looked like armour for a battle.

The shouts, slams and bangs of Mum and the man flew overhead, settled on my shoulders and caused me to sink until I was submerged and underwater and I was trying to wave at them back on land but they couldn't see me, wouldn't notice me. I wondered if I'd died, if my body had been taken by the sea, or just my mind.

A hand reached out to save me, was offering me help, salvation – the clear liquid in the glass I was being handed by my mum pulled me out. She was in the dining room once more, throwing open the door to the cabinet that we stored the booze in for Christmas – bought bit by bit over the year, saved and stored painstakingly – emptying it out frantically. Then she was back. This time the liquid was brown. Then red. I kept swallowing as directed, taking what was good for me, even when it was rejected and hit the roof of my mouth coming back up from where it had just landed. I kept swallowing,

85

gasping for air, being saved, even when I was sure I was being killed.

That night was the night of my first blackout. I don't remember putting down the glass, saying goodnight, walking up the stairs away from their continuing screams, going to the toilet, wiping between my legs, taking off my trousers, taking off my top, putting on my nightie, getting into bed and closing my eyes. But I must have done those things, or at least some of them, just like I did every night.

My mum woke me just before seven a.m. for my shift in the café in town where I was a £1.88-an-hour Saturday girl. I heard her voice saying my name, telling me to get up, coming at me from far away, somewhere I couldn't initially see or reach. When it finally did arrive, it was coupled with nausea, which distracted from the pain of the grip on my skull, the handle slowly turning, the nuts, the bolts tightening, closing the gaps in the cracks. I rode the bus to work, clutched my insides in place over every bump. I'd barely got my white apron tied at the base of my back with a bow before I was throwing up on the cobbles of the alley out back. As I spat on the stone, watching what I thought had saved me running downhill into the pavement cracks while trying to avoid the splashback of sick on my shoes, I knew that drinking wasn't for me, however much I lusted after oblivion. The lack of control. The primal forces that took over my body when it was forced to vomit against my will: stomach tightened, mouth open, teeth bared as whatever was in my gut hurtled up through my throat and out into the air with zero cooperation from me. Eyes bulged, fists gripped, muscles stiffened as my body fought what it must do. I vowed: drinking wasn't for me. A vow that I was to keep for several years – touching barely a drop, never ever more than three drinks in one night – until I discovered that, actually, drinking was very much for me.

CHAPTER 11

Our house always felt sticky with sex, with lust. It was in the fabric of the carpet, the paint on the walls, always hanging in the air. I knew that Mum was attractive, that men found her sexy. Lots of men. 'They say I've got the best bum in the village,' she'd say with a smile.

Saturday night. She'd allow me to be her confidante, her friend, from the moment she ran her bath. I sat on the toilet and talked to her as the water and foam gently lapped her breasts, which had settled down next to her armpits. As I got older, I knew that women's bodies were meant to curve in and out in specific places and that, when that happened, men would like you and want to be with you.

I remember times when she called to me, got me to hook her into her stockings and suspenders, worn under her leather skirt on the nights she seemed happiest. After she got dressed, she would be in the kitchen, head down, blow-drying her permed blonde hair until it was big enough, spraying its bombast into place.

Those were the best nights. The house became slowly infused with new smells, warmth, hustle and bustle. The sharp edges softened, became buttery. It began when the immersion heater was switched on – a very rare treat. We were under strict instructions to use it only in an emergency – we couldn't afford it – though I was never quite sure what would constitute an emergency. As the water in the tank tucked into the corner of my bedroom started to simmer, then bubble and boil, Mum's excitement levels rose.

The kitchen smelled of bubble bath and Elnett and perfume and make-up. She was scarlet-cheeked with excitement and optimism. Anything could happen after she exited the door and was free from us, from that house. I knew that it was this that flooded her eyes with light, that pressed the switch inside her. The nights when she was not our mum, she was just Jane.

It started to become clear to me how suffocated she felt by motherhood, by us. Her identity permanently erased before she'd properly been able to form her own. If you become a mother at sixteen, you're barely an adult, barely a person. Sister, daughter, now wife and mother. When did she get to be her own woman? Every time she looked at us, she was reminded of what she'd sacrificed, lost, never ever had.

I looked at my own body as it changed, and felt so far away from being a woman, *that* kind of woman. I was plonked onto the dining-room chair, a stained towel around my shoulders, as she undid the boxes that contained perming lotion and bleach. She worked away to put my hair in permanent tight, tight curls and paint it with streaks of yellow. The end of the plastic hook dug into my skull while it retrieved strands of hair for her to stain. I knew I was nothing to look at; I felt she wanted me to look better than I did naturally. And under her hands, as I sensed her stare shifting to something edging towards approval, it seemed like I was becoming someone people might look at. That people might actually see.

Men liked Mum, liked what they saw when they looked at her. And it seemed as though there were always men in our house. Sometimes they'd be there for years, other times months. Sometimes weeks, nights, hours. The men my mum beckoned over the threshold came in every shape, every size, type, taste. There were lovers, boyfriends, fiancés, friends and husbands – both other people's and her own.

Mum's speciality appeared to be men who shouldn't be there, who would pay the price for coming over. Who would turn up, invited, in the middle of the day. I remember walking in the back door and hearing a man grunting. Headboards and floorboards banged. I slammed a door to let them know that I was home, that – Christ, anyway, it was only 3.30 p.m. The men who were there at strange hours were oftentimes men I knew. A man whose wife eventually rang the house and told me to tell Mum to leave her husband alone. The men parked their cars at the bottom of our street, letting the world know that they were there to knock on number ten's door.

I can recall no formal introduction (or any other kind) to those who stuck around in the morning – there would just be a strange man walking down the stairs. They all seemed to stink of booze and fags and look at us like we were intruding, even though it was our home. They were at home immediately, boots under the table. They filled the entire sofa in the front room, took charge of the remote control, filled the house with smoke and rage. Faces appeared hard against us, three children they didn't want, but made peace with accepting so they could be with Mum, for however long or short a time that might be. In the morning, they eyed us warily, seemingly wondering in the cold light of day if they had made the right choice. Wondering whether there was another option, whether we were really around for good, whether we were really immovable. When they were gone, when it was just us again, I breathed. I exhaled. I wished, prayed, elbows apart, for there to be no more men. But just days, weeks later they were back again and it was no longer only us. And I felt a new kind of terror in familiar skin inside our house.

As a teenager, I felt ashamed, dirty by association. How could Mum do this to me? How could she do this to other women? To children? I hated her with a violence and fever I didn't know I was capable of. She disgusted me. It seemed to me that she gave away her body too easily to men who weren't hers, men whom she couldn't always name.

As an extension of my hatred for her, I hated myself.

I became obsessed with how much I hated my face. Not the kind of flippant, lightly held hate that occasionally irritated and wrinkled the skin. But the kind that was felt constantly: when it wasn't burning right behind your eyes turning them red, it was sitting in the pit of your stomach, swilling and swirling, lapping against your insides, corroding them with each backwash. I never, ever didn't feel it. And even though I barely recognised my own face, I still hated it. Each time I caught a glimpse in a window, a mirror, sliced in the back of a fork, I was shocked anew. Surprised by the circle of flesh looking back. Who was she? What was she? Sometimes, no matter how hard I looked, I simply wasn't there to see. There was just nothing. These were also my favourite times.

When I could, I would lock myself in the bathroom, both desperate and unwilling to spend some time getting to know my own face. I stood in front of the mirror set into the cabinet screwed into the wall. I traced the outline of my own face with my fingers and thumbs. Running from my hairline at my forehead down both sides, past my ears, around and under my chin, up over my nose and eyelids until I was back where I started. Taking one flat hand, I ran it over my skull, traversing the raised bump made of bone and flesh that had sat there since I couldn't remember when. Then, courage summoned, I headed for the bit I hated the most. The three moles that sat in an almost perfect triangle across my face. One on the right between my mouth and chin, two on the left: one tucked between my nose and my upper lip, the other by the bottom. I ran a single finger over them, feeling their tougher outline. They made me feel physically sick. The brown dots stuck on my face. The reason I kept my head down, always faced the floor, was terrified of looking anyone directly in the face. I took the face-pack sample I'd found in the back of the cabinet, squeezed the white paste out onto my fingers and smeared it as thickly as camouflage paint onto my face.

I began with the moles, dabbing on top of the brown until it was gone. Mesmerised by the simple beauty of my face without them, I kept going further and further from the brown, smearing the white wider and higher, wider and higher until I reached my ears, my hairline, my neck. I looked in the mirror, my nose, cheeks, chin, all features obliterated. I looked so beautiful, finally.

CHAPTER 12

Getting away was the only possible solution. The furthest place away from home I knew was London – and the only way I could think of to get there was by going to university. The first person in my family to stay in education after sixteen, I was met with rolled eyes at home and the assertion that 'we can't afford to support you'. Fuck it: I was going.

I spent the years before leaving home for good holding myself together – barely – by my fingertips. Home was still a battlefield. I was weary. After we ended up in emergency accommodation without beds or hot water, on an estate far rougher than ours, while the latest bad marriage behind the door of number ten was imploding, I went to live with my glorious nana.

My focus was laser-sharp: I had to pass my exams. I needed to get the fuck out of there as soon as I could. I counted off each minute, each hour, each day: silent, steadfast. Holding my hopes, my dreams, close to my chest. I didn't dare reveal what I wanted to anyone else, terrified they would take it away from me. But I knew that if I didn't leave, I'd die there. In between the cracks and fractures I'd fall, into nothingness.

The same focus propelled me through university, then down to London. By the time I arrived, just weeks after my final exam, to start my job as a magazine PA, the determination was being replaced by anger. I was, to my surprise, perpetually furious. I was consumed by an anger that made me pink, made me tremble. Why me? I raged. Of course, the real question was: why not me? But I imagined my life otherwise: I saw the woman I could have become, if I hadn't been changed, marked forever. Nothing could ever make me clean, make me like new. He – the first of the two of my mum's boyfriends to sexually abuse me – had broken me, right there under the light of the moon, and every night when I saw it rise and set, I saw once more what and who I was, irrevocably. What and who those hands, in those hours, had shaped me into. And I hated him for all of it. I hated the moon for all of it. And more than either, I hated myself for every last tiny bit of it.

The men who came after broke me in different ways – with their fists, with their words. They called me stupid, pathetic, nobody. I willed myself into invisibility, kept silent, kept still, tried to be the nothing that they were so sure I was. But inside, the voices were loud. My fight was simply being stored for a safer time. It looked like I'd shrunk, curled up inside myself, but I hadn't done it with passivity and compliance. I'd done it with patient fury – a coiled spring, waiting for release.

That fury became something I couldn't control. I persuaded myself that I had a handle on it. I called it strength. I called it fortitude. But it circulated throughout my body, making me not just hard, but brittle. In the end I decided that there was only one way to sate the rage fizzing against my gums. To fix what the man who had stolen me from myself had done.

As I worked for a media company, I now had access to the electoral roll. All I had to do was send a name and a town to the woman who ran the library and I had an address in return. She had no idea that I was going to use that address to find and kill him.

He lived just six miles away from our village, in the centre of town. I memorised the address, could see his road, house, the street light outside. I planned what I was going to do. What would happen when I visited him. I would arrive in his town, wait until the sky blackened, the street quietened, night fell. I would walk down the street, slowly, arrive at this gate, lift the latch, walk through, close it and – quietly yet firmly – let the latch lock.

I would knock on his door; he'd open it, look at me and know who and what I was. My body, my brain dug up from beneath the soil he'd thrown and patted down over my head. He thought I was buried. He thought I was dead. He thought he'd been the end of me: his cock, his fingers, the whispers in his mouth murdering me. I'd lain dead and buried for twenty years, but now I'd come to find him, to get my revenge. To watch him twist and turn and break. In that moment, he'd know why I was there, why I'd come looking for him. That he was the one about to die, about to be buried, my name escaping his bleeding lips as brown soil filled his mouth and choked my name out of him.

We'd go inside, and I'd tell him: *nothing you did touched me; your attempts to destroy my life, at the age of five, were for nothing. I've always been stronger, harder, braver than you.* He would gasp and panic for breath, for the words to make it all OK. He'd try to work out what could possibly save him in the coming seconds, minutes. And while his mind raced, his fingers jerked and retracted, I'd pick up the bat and swing it at his head.

The first thwack would be the single most satisfying, pleasing sound I'd ever have heard. The sound of wood meeting bone, specifically skull. It would crack on impact, fracturing and piercing his brain. Blood, brain, leaking out into the space between his mind and his head, sloshing around like a baby in a bath. He'd be on his knees as I took the bat to both arms, his hips, the ribs. I'd take a knife and stick it into the white expanse of his throat. It'd lodge and stick and I'd pull with both hands: down, across, blood spurting, gushing out as he tried to scream, tried to stop the wound, but could only mouth silently while his flapping hands jammed inside his open throat and he impaled himself on his own fist, his body jerking and bucking under the weight.

I'd stand over him, watching the last twitches and spasms of his body in his final moments, as he clasped and grabbed at my feet and ankles, smearing blood all over me. I would look deep into his eyes as he died, the light fading from his big brown eyes until they were empty and flat. I would step over him and leave his house exactly as I entered, the blood under my feet creating a trail out of the door and down the street.

Those who came to try to rescue him and who would later bury him would know that I was there. Or someone like me. That he had done something so brutal, so beyond forgiveness and understanding that I had no option but to end him like he ended me. I had to end what he started all those years ago. And for me to live, to survive, he had to die.

CHAPTER 13

The rage blossomed, touched the far reaches of me. I had believed that all I needed was to reach London and my life would be OK; *I* would be OK. But it hadn't worked out like that. What few gaps were left untouched by rage were filled with sadness. And I needed to get it out of me.

I lay in the dry, empty white bath, ran the water, splashing over and around my skin, until it filled up around me. I left the cold tap untouched; the water that gushed and flowed over me scalded my skin a deep, livid red, the colour of poppies in November.

I took the plastic lady razor in my hands, captivated by the promise of what lay ahead. I hadn't yet learnt to smash the razor out of its plastic casing, so it was a much harder, bloodier job. I took shallow breaths, held it in my right hand, lifted my thigh and an arm out of the water. I placed the razor against my skin, gritted my teeth, swallowed, shut my eyes tight and yanked down, across, as hard as I could. It pared me open and blood spilled out of the slices and onto my skin and down into the bath water, which became pink and cloudy right up to my neck. I put my head beneath the surface of water, mouth open and dark in the diluted iron I was floating in.

The monsters were inside me. The one monster. I felt him beneath the covers; I saw the shape of him at night, felt the touch of him on my sliced skin. I broke beneath him all over again, our bones blended together until I couldn't see where he ended and I began. We were the same person; he'd had hold of me for almost all of my life. But I hadn't realised it, thought I had relegated him to the shadows. And now he was back to claim what was his: me. The thread that had been left on the floor as a little girl, he'd picked up in both hands and made it into rope for me. I drank every night, picked up a cheap bottle of red from the local shop and skipped food altogether. My obsession with hurting myself grew and grew.

I'd been involved with a new man, older than me, who seemed to know me absolutely and not at all. He thought I was mad; I *was* mad. I called him over and over, desperate to be told we were OK, but really that I was OK. I would wake up of a morning, not really sure what I'd done the night before. I went out, drank too much, woke in the early hours to go to the toilet and found the entire bathroom painted in bright red vomit – it was in the sink, on the ceiling, on the door, on the toilet. I got on my hands and knees to clean it up and by the time daylight came I couldn't remember if it was ever there or if it had been a violent night-mare.

The days and the nights passed in the same high-pitched frequency. I walked from one room, one street, to another, never really knowing where I was, who I was. I barely registered the people I passed as I did. Whether I knew them or not. The thick layer between me and the world numbed me, kept me safe, but isolated me entirely. Inside the white warmth, I slowly went more mad. I couldn't sleep, except for when I was unconscious from drinking. I became deranged. I stockpiled pills, painkillers from over the counter and emptied them into a drawer. I texted the man and my mum to say that I loved them. The first handful went down the hardest. The tablets were dry, my swallow tentative, scared. The cheap red wine added a layer of roughage to the pills, made my throat close and gag.

Once the first fistful was out of the way, the second, the third, the fourth were easier. I drank and drank the very bad wine. I lay on the bed, waiting for the gradual drift-off that I'd seen, read about. But I just felt sad, mad and sick. I was sick in my own mouth and swallowed it down. I played the same song over and over, the repetition like the car that went round and round the block soothing the baby.

Then, banging. The shout of 'Fire Brigade'. I stayed perfectly still, presuming that I could make them disappear by willing it so.

They started to try to break the door down. The banging got louder; the rhythmic booming calmed me. Fifteen minutes later, the door had still not given way, and they were not giving up. There seemed to be no other way out. I went downstairs to my flatmate's room. She had so far slept through the many men trying to crash through the front door below.

'There are some people who want to get in,' I said.

She looked at me, in my underwear, cuts showing, crying, and she finally heard the banging. Then she was up, on her feet, and there were people, people, people. They wanted to know what I'd taken; they were not so bothered about why. I'd taken the paracetamol tablets. My skin had come out in hives. I'd turned red all over and couldn't stop crying. They asked about my cuts. I told everyone that *I just wanted to die.*

When I got to the hospital they told me that I could have died, that if I'd just gone to sleep I would have done – not immediately, beautifully, serenely – but later, once the paracetamol had eaten my liver and other organs. Then it would have been too late. They gave me an IV drip. The man came; he brought a book of poetry called *Staying Alive.* He left and I didn't see him again.

Someone, I'm not sure who, apparently called my mum. She didn't jump in a car, onto a train. She stayed at home. Said there was nothing she could do anyway. Then, by surreal coincidence, her friend overdosed on insulin a few hours later. She went to her bedside. She called me afterwards on the hospital phone and said, 'How can people be so selfish as to do that to themselves?' I agreed.

She didn't come that night or at all. I woke up the next morning and my best friend, who'd been in Manchester, was sitting at the end of my bed. My eyes filled with tears at this moment of extraordinary kindness, a kindness I wasn't used to and struggled to recognise.

The nurses changed shift and the new one stopped by my bed, examined the IV and my notes and tutted, 'I thought so.' Apparently I looked like the kind of girl who would try to commit suicide.

I was due to go home the next day, but the psychiatrist I'd seen once since being admitted needed to speak to me. The man and my flatmate had been to see her. They told her that they didn't think I was well enough to go home. My flatmate said she was convinced that she'd come home to find me hanged from a noose off the ceiling. I was livid. How dare she expose me to them?

The doctor suggested that I stay in the hospital. I refused. She mentioned sectioning. I argued against it. I lied beautifully. I wasn't suicidal; I'd never *really* been suicidal. I hadn't even really been depressed. I'd just been having a hard time. I talked my way out of it. She let me go home. My friend's dad came down. He made dinner, put food in the oven, talked to me about life and what it meant, ultimately, and I was so desperately sad and grateful for this act, I thought my heart might stop right there and then.

But it still felt like it was just the first act. That it wasn't over. That the shadow would be back to claim me again. I waited for him.

CHAPTER 14

I'm sitting in Heathrow. It's May 2012. I have a slight pile of dollars – ending my life in London had pretty much entirely cleared me out – and a copy of *American Psycho*. That and one giant pink plastic Primark suitcase is all I have with which to start my new life in New York, where I've taken a job on a magazine.

I sit outside W.H. Smith, my legs frozen at the thought of walking to the gate. I want to go; I *really* do. I think. But I have a weight in my stomach that won't shift. A rock lassoed with rope and tied to the bottom of my rib cage. Every movement reminds me that it's there, as I walk down the white corridors, along the moving metal pathways and arrive at the gate. The plane's there. Once I step onto that plane, I know it's all going to change. Everything.

I clutch my tote bag and handbag tight. When I get up, too quickly, jerking as they call out the row number my ears have been listening for, my fingers flex open and both of my bags fly through the air and land at the feet of a suited man who glances at me with thinly veiled irritation. Heat and colour rush to my face and *I'm so, so sorry*, on my knees, pushing two-pence pieces and bits of torn-up paper, red lipsticks without lids and tampons that have no wrappers back inside the bags. As I kneel among the mess of the life I am not really leaving behind, but carrying on with me, I remind myself that I don't believe in signs and, if I did, I certainly wouldn't believe in one as heavy-handed as this.

The plane takes off and the zooming, zapping excitement, the kind that is supposed to crash through your bloodstream and into your bones at moments like this, is absent. I muster up a touch of fear, an emotion I'm innately more comfortable with, asking for wine, hoping that this will prove to be the kindling for the feelings I've misplaced. Possibly never had.

I arrive in New York, knowing that the answer to everything, the way to fill the gaps inside me, is on the other side of the Arrivals gate. I get in the line for a yellow taxi and then I'm in the back.

Speeding speeding speeding speeding.

The skyline comes into view, the one that I've dreamed of, fantasised about, touched and tasted in films, in books. The lights, the noise, the fever I beckon into my open ears. In the middle of the skyline, the Empire State Building rises, her majesty cutting through the cotton clouds, her mystery, her seduction in full flow.

Before I'd ever even set foot on the hot pavement, the city was burned on my brain. Not just what it looked like, but what I thought it felt like. From the Brooklyn

106

brownstones and the Manhattan rooftops to the steaming manholes and the glittering skyline: I'd seen it and experienced it thousands of times over.

Whenever stress made my shoulders sag or I shared sour words with a friend, I'd escape to that bit of my brain marked 'New York' and wander the streets there, feeling free. I knew that the city was not only holding the life I'd been waiting to live, but the best version of me I was still set to be.

Yet, now, here, my body in the place it had longed to be in, I feel cold and underwhelmed, unmoved. My stomach stays in place, static. I stare out of the window, waiting, willing myself to feel . . . something. I have to. How else is the city going to carve me out anew?

The cab pulls up at the apartment I'm staying at – a tiny, neat Airbnb on the Lower East Side between a Chinese take-out and a dry cleaning store. From the window of the perfectly square white kitchen, with its perfectly round white table and two matching chairs, it has a view uptown, of the Empire State. To the right of the kitchen sits an efficient two-seater sofa, in what could never really be described, truly, as a living room. Then right again lies a green bathroom, with a bath built out of tiles, and a plastic divider rising out of the edges of the bath to protect whatever modesty might be on display. Through the final door lies a bedroom with a bed close to the floor on slats, and a TV on the wall dominating the room.

I know from their Airbnb bio that a PR girl lives here

with her boyfriend, apart from the times they rent it out for fistfuls of quick cash. I try to glean clues of their existence from the flat, which is spick and span, precise and controlled. There's no room between the furniture and the walls. Your movement is dictated entirely by the shape of the apartment and the objects that have been placed in it, mapping your way. Could they not dance in the kitchen if they feel like dancing? Where do they hold each other? Where do they laugh?

I walk out of the flat and go to the bar on the corner, sit on a high stool at the bar and order a pint of beer from a weary bartender, scratching his beard. I imagine that, hearing my accent, the other person at the bar – a dark-haired man in jeans deliberately designed to look dirty, and a leather jacket – will turn to me and ask me about myself. This is how New York will go for me. How it goes for everyone when they arrive. He doesn't look up from his phone. There are a handful of couples in the bar – a bar that I will come to know well. None of them glance my way.

For a second I wonder if I'm invisible. Do I exist here? With these people? I watch them talking, touching hands, fingers, elbows lightly. A brunette with black-rimmed glasses and a single tattoo laughs. The Strokes play. I feel like I've walked onto a stage play where they've just finished blocking out the painted scenery, a member of the audience who's taken a wrong turn and ended up in the middle of the action, against all the rules, ruining all the work that has already been done.

Disrupting the flow. I drink. Stepping outside, the world shifts around me and wobbles, waves coming over the Williamsburg Bridge. The yellow traffic lights are perfectly in position, the rectangular street signs nestling next to each other, pointing off in different directions, like an air traffic controller bringing us, them, home. Yellow taxis, horns honking, a bodega cat arching its back in the doorway, trash on the street corner already rotting and spewing itself into the air, the cigarette smoke that billows and jets past, carried along on a thin-legged stride.

The familiar and alien jostle and jut against each other. My head swims and I close my eyes, astonished that the picture, the stage remains set when I open them. I walk the block and a half back to the apartment, a performative walk. I feel I'm being watched, being assessed. I get into bed, even though it's not yet dark, I turn on the TV and lie under the covers as the commercials rush through the adverse side effects of whatever medicine is being sold: *heart attack, excessive sweating, impotence, baldness, rash, blisters, stroke, high cholesterol, high blood pressure, kidney failure, cancer, coma, death.*

My first week at work begins the next morning. The sense of otherness and emptiness has followed me from the apartment to the office I sit in. I look out through the one window onto the floor at the people whose heads barely pivot to mine. The hours drag and contort in front of my eyes. I feel as if I'm on display; they watch to see what I'll do, how I act. Every arm stretch for the phone, every word scribbled down, feels contrived, unreal.

Most of the women I'm working with have been excruciatingly rude and unfriendly so far — a highlight is being told 'I won't stab you in the back, I'll stab you in the front' on my first day. Several of them wanted my job, it would seem, and are furious they didn't get it. Conversations end when I enter a room. Direct questions are ignored, no matter how many times I ask.

I go to the bathroom. I want to disappear, if only for a second. There's no toilet seat on the bowl and I sit cross-legged on the floor, my hands clasped over my ears so I can lock the world out, enjoy the muffling and the woolly noise.

I'm not sure how long I'm in there, but it's long: too long. The lights turn off, presumably because I'm not moving, my muscles tense and hold, my hands still and tight over my head. I sit in the dark and feel terrified. I become convinced that someone has turned the lights off and is waiting outside for me to emerge, feeling my way, delivering myself into their hands, their patient violence.

My breath quickens and deepens, the tingle reaching my limbs, my head, as I sit like a statue, frozen and taut. Seconds pass, minutes pass as I sit there; I'm not sure how many. Tears start to run down my face as I try to stay completely still, completely quiet.

Then, *whoosh*, the bathroom door opens and light floods the room once more. I take my hands from over my ears, open my eyes, stand up, straighten my skirt, pull two sheets of tissue from the dispenser and wipe my face before walking out, face contorted into something approaching, if not a smile, then a non-grimace. I go back to my desk and it continues.

CHAPTER 15

Two weeks later, on what is, I'll come to learn, a typical New York summer's day, I move into my first proper apartment.

In the ninety-plus-degree Manhattan heat, the sun roasts the foul rubbish that has been heaped out on the sidewalk and kicked around: scraps of meat cooking for the second time, now moist and sticking underfoot. Horns scream, steam charges, sweat runs into the cracks of cement between the bricks that make the buildings that hold the sky that puts a lid on the madness bubbling and bursting out down below.

The advert describes a large studio with charming period features: an enviable location in the famous, infamous Greenwich Village, on Christopher Street. The place where all of the artists and weirdos and outsiders and beautiful freaks I carry inside me had lived, had walked, before my feet brought me here in the shadow of theirs.

Up the stairs, the stairs, the stairs, the stairs, the stairs, past the sticky off-white walls, over rough grey carpets, there is a chipped grey door. Inside the door: one room, two windows on the farthest wall that look out onto more windows, more bricks. A tree looms, the shadows of its branches lying across the bed, casting a stain across the body that lies there, never moving.

The kitchen has no windows, no light, save for the harsh yellow bulb in the ceiling that glints off the chef's knives lining the wall as they wait, waiting for me and my gasping, thirsty skin. A couch and an old TV are the only landmarks between them and the bed. A thin rectangular room is tucked behind a door holding a burnt orange bathroom, a toilet that will block often and an exposed pipe connected to a makeshift shower.

Across the hall, two grey doors identical to mine, just with different numbers. One is vibrating, pulsating, shuddering under the sound of the shrieking, moaning, screaming women of the violent porn being played on a loop inside by a man whose face I will never see, not once, in the year to come. I think of him often, I think of the women on his screen, who need me, who need rescuing from him.

I pay $2,500 for a shoebox, surrounded by other people existing in their own shoeboxes. The ten-feet by thirty-feet rectangles holding us all inside our own stories, our own dreams, our own nightmares. The sounds, smells, tastes slipping underneath the doors and out into the world we keep at bay, the small clues to what is really happening in every apartment, in every room, in every building, on every street, in every neighbourhood, higher and tighter and more and more until the breath is taken from us and we stand tall, sucking the few inches of air above our heads.

I email a friend:

'So here I am in New York. Here I am, alone. All alone.'

I didn't know then what alone truly means. It's more than being a new arrival in a city, without familiar colleagues, without friends, without people to call your own, people who call you theirs. I will learn though.

I've cut off my British phone – deliberately, so that I can't be reached by who and what I've left behind. My ex-boyfriend who, just a handful of months before had told me, in an email, about his new girlfriend, their new home and then just weeks later, a follow-up about their new baby. His news had me dry-heaving and spitting into the office toilet as another woman pissed long and hard in the cubicle next to me.

Their new family – formed just days after I arrive in the city, with their son's birth – couldn't reach me if I didn't have a phone to receive pictures and updates from concerned friends who just want to check if I have seen the pictures on the internet and if I haven't I shouldn't, absolutely under any circumstances, go looking for them.

For three weeks the only place I have internet or telephone access is at work and I feel protected, hardened by the isolation, the complete absence of life, or any kind of love, that I recognise.

My birthday comes around; I turn thirty-three alone

on my knees on the floor of my apartment. The splinters burrow into my scarred kneecaps as I kneel. I cry, beg, claw the walls, the floors. I'm bleeding as my hands face each other and come together.

That first summer, I dye my hair fire-engine red. I cut my fringe into a hard, high line. I'll soon dye it dark brown. And then I'll dye it black. I can't remember what I used to look like, what she used to look like just a handful of weeks before. I look at pictures from before and see the woman I was, smiling, the light almost reaching her eyes, feel her between my fingers and in my mind. Her hair is yellow and her eyes are blue and she looks happy and free and light as air and I touch her, touch her almost-happiness. It bubbles and bites. I pull back. I'm too far away now.

I go to places with other people in them, in search of her. I look for her yellow, brittle strands, the bursting bright blue. In the places where men buy me drinks because I'm alone reading Jay McInerney. In the bar in the French restaurant half a block away where no one buys the glass after glass I drink. Before I can't remember anything, I remember telling the soft-eyed owner about being lonely, about feeling so very sad. The record store with the two short aisles bursting with old British magazines, browning around the edges, and old records slipped into thick plastic. I feel them between fingers that shake a little now, the ends chewed and torn and the brightest pink, striped, lashed with red. I feel at home; I can touch it. The dust slips inside the small areas of exposed skin and I smear it in my broken hair and I'm here and I don't feel like drinking or diving or dying or going somewhere else. I can see straight, briefly.

Those seconds, those minutes, are not the seconds and minutes that make up the hours that make up my days. I wander from place to place, drink to drink, until the grey becomes black and I'm swallowed and get home God knows how and every morning when I wake up, I'm always surprised, sometimes crestfallen, to have been spat out again, tender and bruised and somehow a little less than when I was sucked up.

But at night, it's the coat I wear, tugged around me, that I hate taking off, refuse to. It comes with me everywhere. It becomes my skin. My blood, my hair, my teeth, my touch, my taste.

Within weeks, I have a list of bars I'd rather not visit, some that I simply can't from sheer embarrassment and shame. The number of blocks I have to walk to get a drink in safety, with dignity, growing alongside it. There's too much chance of recognition, specifically things I don't want to be recognised for.

On the good nights, I lose things: my favourite faux fur coat, my red leather gloves, my passport, my bank card, my phone. On the bad nights, I lose more: chunks of my memory, all the feeling in my hands and toes, my loosening hold on my sanity.

On the nights in between, I fight with the bartender about the jukebox ('Why did you fucking skip New Order? Give me my five dollars back!'). I climb on the hood of a parked car, knees flinching, fighting against the cold, hard metal. Lying on my back, looking at the sky with drunken terror. I let a man whose face never comes into focus kiss me badly against the jukebox as The Smiths play, his hands pulling my mascara and eyeliner down my face in black stripes, tyre tracks from the hit and run. On those nights, my eyes are ringed, hollow, sunk in black; the bright red of my lipstick is smeared up to where my cheekbone hits my eye socket. My reflection is that of a stranger. A clown.

And on the very bad nights, the worst ones, there's mess to be cleared up the next day. A mind to be patched up, a body to be fixed, a memory to be erased, if it was ever captured in the first place. A scientist once told me that when you reach a certain level of drunkenness, your brain stops recording events. So, the next morning, what you think has been forgotten, what you desperately try to retrieve, simply isn't there, never has been, never will be. I cling to this in the moments that I rummage for drunken memories in the wreckage of my nights, my days. They don't exist. And in those moments, I reason, neither do I.

I like drinking. Very much. Or rather, I like what drinking does to me. I like feeling altered. Very much. I like feeling the mundanity and misery of normality dissolve under my tongue. The anxiety that balls my fists, locks my shoulders, fixes my grin disappears. My body loosens, my mind softens, clouds drift in and the release feels like escape.

The mornings are impossible. Every morning is impossible. The ritual cripples me. Wake up, panic, feel guilty and/or ashamed, vomit, shower, vomit (sometimes in the shower), dress, paint my face, pour drops in my eyes to dissolve away the lightning streaks and shoots of red.

Weekends are the worst; my mornings, days, free of the commitment to be somewhere, to be somebody. I never, ever dare make any plans for a Saturday or Sunday; I know that I will likely be unconscious until the afternoon. The freedom means I drink longer, more heavily, with even more enthusiasm than usual. I wake up and vomit – the only part of my weekday routine that I carry over – before taking to the couch where I sleep, eat delivery food, vomit some more and watch TV until it's time to do it all again. This isn't the consequence of nights of fun and abandon: I'm usually alone – definitely by the end of the night if not at the start. I don't need company to drink and my drinking means that many people don't want to be in my company. Which works out well all round.

I become obsessed with booze: when can I start drinking, what will happen when that half-full bottle is emptied, why has no one ordered another yet, can I order another drink yet? I start to sneak by the bar at any moments that present themselves – shots of liquor swallowed at gigs and restaurants when I'm on my way back from the toilet. At bars when they go out for a smoke. I deliberately don't keep track of my drinks and really hope that no one else does either. There is no greater relief than the change of a bartender shift: the clean slate that comes with a paid bar bill and a pair of eyes that hasn't seen your sliding disposition.

But the more I drink, these people, wherever I am, could be my people. This could be my home. I could be anywhere. I could be comfortable. I could even be happy. At some point, I stop experiencing the night in real time. It becomes a series of memories that I'll revisit or abandon later, carrying some with me home, allowing others to fall away, never ever to be claimed. And at some point in the night, the tape simply, suddenly, runs out.

More and more, I squat in the room with no windows and no light that makes me want to sink and disappear inside its walls. Some days I disassociate completely – I can see the world through the glass dome that I'm suffocating inside, but I can't touch it, feel it, taste it, suck it into my lungs. When I've drifted so far away from myself, I feel that my mind is lost forever, that I'll never make it back to my body. That the loose tie holding it tight has snapped and can never be mended. Those are the worst moments of all, the moments when I know my only option is through the window, my body splattering on the pavement.

A friend mentions Xanax to me: how it soothes, blunts the edges; how everyone takes it. I go to the doctor and before I've even half-finished my story of half-truths ('I feel kinda anxious, I suppose. No big deal, but something to help would be great!'), he is writing a script that says yes, I too can have Xanax. I slip the tiny pink pill, and then a second, onto my tongue. I wait. Twenty minutes later, I feel a soft wave wash over me. Thirty minutes after that, I'm not worrying about anyone, anything. I lie on the bed and watch the outline of the trees outside dance across the ceiling and down the walls. I feel . . . OK. A revolutionary state.

I'm kept moving from point to point by my friends who come to visit, each one sustaining me until the next. Dave is coming to town for the US release of his book. I've offered to let him stay with me, but the reality of what that looks like looms large. I've done a pretty good job of keeping the reality of my New York life from everyone at home so far. But however good an act I put on, he'd *see* the reality. Of me, of where I live. The huge gap between what I am and what I claim to be. He is due to step right slap bang into the middle of it, looking at me in surprise as the water rises past his knees.

He's sleeping on my sofa – brown, dusty – facing the old grey television, dark kitchen to his left, my bed and the only sources of light to his right. I can tell when he arrives that this isn't what he expects, what anyone expects. I make a joke about the lack of windows, the burnt orange walls that always make it look like it's being frozen in time while being burned down from the inside out.

Night one: I join him in the bar where he's reading

an excerpt from his book. I make myself a promise: two drinks, no more. I'll stay sober; I'll stay sane, no matter what. I know no one at the bar, bury my head in my phone, back against the wall. Dave steps up to read under two white, bright lights – charming, funny, already so much more at home in my town within twenty-four hours than I am. Outside the window, they're projecting his face reading, the slight lisp and his British song captivating the whole room of cool, hot, also charming, also funny locals. Some are wearing hats. There's a photographer kneeling just metres away from his knees, capturing this moment. His face hovers twenty feet to my left out of the window. I stay long enough to be polite, until he's finished, then abandon my second drink with half a finger left in the glass and leave. In the cab, I cry. Partly from joy and pride for him. Partly because the thick loneliness has doubled in size. He's been embraced by the city as I stand on the outside, palms against the glass.

The second night: his launch party. Drinks at an apartment in Chelsea owned by another author from his publisher. I know that this will be harder. The opportunities to stand alone, fade into the shadows on the walls, are fewer. I'm buzzed in and stand in the stairwell, paralysed with anxiety, before heading up to the front door. I take two Xanax and then decide to take a third to be on the safe side. The last one tastes bitter as it gets stuck under my tongue.

The fellow author opens the door and I recognise

him. He's a local in the bar downstairs, the bar that I go to a lot, alone. I mentally scan, as quickly as possible, the Rolodex of evenings flashing through my mind. *What has he seen? What have I done?* A brief flash of something — recognition, horror, confusion, Christ knows — flashes across his face, a brief look up and down, before he straightens it out, the impeccable host, and welcomes me inside, with the half sweep of a hand (it was a Manhattan apartment, after all).

Inside, over and around him, there are floating heads, perfectly round. The room is about a third full of small people, all dressed in black and brown, a statistically impossible amount in glasses. They're talking in three tiny, tight pockets, cradling small drinks on white paper napkins that are perfectly square. I look from one to the other, feeling naked.

I spot Dave with relief.

'Terri's come as a cartoon character,' he says. The group pauses. One laughs, one swallows drily, one looks away, another coughs.

I laugh — 'You know me!' — and smooth down my creased dress that I haven't had time to iron. I can see how I look, what they must see. My broken hair, pinned high and tight. Scarlet slash of a mouth. Tight reproduction 1950s wiggle dress — blue with white trim. Cherry-red stilettos are cutting the feet that curl up inside them.

I walk to the kitchen and help myself to a drink. I drink it fast; there's another. I do what feels like the most unnatural act in the world and walk into an almost closed circle of people already talking. They warily make a few inches for me to stand in and continue talking while I nod, one hand holding another drink, the other gripping the forearm with all my might to keep me present, to stop me smashing up everything around me while I scream.

I see the alternative events unloading in my mind as I nod, smile, make *uh-huh* noises. Eventually, manners kick in. They ask me what I do. There's an eye roll at the word 'journalism'. Oh, those magazines, they say, eyebrows raised, foreheads tight.

A mutual friend and his wife arrive, and I take solace with them and the bottle of tequila which someone might have bought or someone might have just found. I remember a shot, two shots and then black.

I wake, fully dressed, on top of my sheets. I roll my tongue over inside my teeth, which are sticky. I can taste, feel, sick. I roll over on my back, grab my phone, see with relief that I'm not late for work, but then I'm hit with instant panic as I realise, know, that Dave isn't there. I look over at the sofa to be sure and it's empty, blanket folded up on top of the single pillow. There's a brick in my chest. I can't remember, but I know something bad happened. I did something bad.

The thing about blackouts is that, more often than not, the memory is gone forever. I spend years and years trying to retrieve them, to fish them out with a hook from the tightest crevices and recesses of my mind. The memory, the exact words and shapes and acts may not be there – what I did with my mouth, my hands, my feet, my legs – but the knowledge that I'd done something, something bad, is always with me. The bit of my brain that decided not to record the memory isn't going to let me off the hook that easily. I carry the stink of shame and embarrassment and panic around with me until I see the place or the person I picked it up.

I call Dave. He answers.

'Where are you?' I ask.

'Do you not remember?'

'No.'

He tells me, matter-of-factly, that I ruined his party. That I got drunk, shouted, I might have cried. That I'd fled and told him he couldn't stay at mine. He'd had to find somewhere else to sleep and is currently in Brooklyn.

Everything gets very still as he talks. I notice dust, the air carrying bits of my skin past me as I stare out of the window. I want to jump through it.

He meets me after work in an Indian restaurant in the Village. I barely taste my food as I apologise over and over, and though he says the right words with considerable grace, he can't meet my eyes. I've never felt more ashamed, hated myself more. The bodies continue to pile up.

CHAPTER 16

It's October when warning comes of the impending Hurricane Sandy – the post-tropical cyclone which will go on to cause the deaths of seventy-one people in America. I have no idea what I'm about to experience or how to prepare for it. I think of soft British winds and scattered showers, and I go to the bodega on the corner and buy supplies: crisps, biscuits, two apples, cakes and two candles. I don't buy booze – I never allow myself to drink at home – a decision I will come to regret. We're sent home early from work just before it's declared unsafe to travel.

I make it home as the wind starts howling with a roar and the rain pounds down. I sit watching events unfold on television, idly flicking between all of the channels showing the same thing. Then: nothing. No noise, no light. The electricity goes out and my apartment is plunged into silent darkness. I start texting friends back in the UK, but a few minutes later, the bars on my cell phone disappear and service goes completely. I go to the toilet and flush, but no water rushes up and out. I try the sink: there's just the squeaking of the taps against the dry spout.

I realise I have no phone reception, no access to email or the internet and no TV. I have no choice but to wait it out, alone, in darkness, as the storm rages on and on outside. For how long, I have no clue. I burn through my two candles in hours, ration out the meagre food. I lie on the bed, in total darkness, the trees outside hurtling towards my windows, never following through on their threat. I make no effort to roll out of their way, just in case the worst happens. The streets outside are empty, pitch-black. The wind picks up papers, trash and takes them careering through the air. I watch them as they dance. I have no clue, at any point, what time it is. With little to do but sleep, I wake not knowing if it's a new day or still the same one, what's dawn and what's sunset.

I hear what I think are voices, chanting, chanting, chanting. Or are they thoughts? I hear them in my dreams and when I'm awake, when the wind blows and the windows rattle and when it's perfectly still. I see shadows curl up and crawl the walls, their body blending with mine on the ceiling.

On what I think is the fourth day, the wind has stopped and I decide to venture outside, hoping it's safe. I feel my way down the stairs of my building in complete darkness, the electricity still off. As I open the door to my building and step outside, I'm relieved to see hand-fuls of people wandering outside, though they looked dazed, confused.

A few of the local stores are selling their remaining stock for cash only, but I have none and the ATMs are down. Everything else is closed – the bars, the restaurants, the liquor stores – and trees and power lines lie crumpled and broken in the streets.

I hear one of the people wandering around aimlessly like me say that there is electricity and cell signal uptown, so I start to walk. And when I hit 34th Street, there it is – half of the city lit up like it's Christmas. My phone springs back to life – amongst the concerned messages, one from a friend from London who is in town.

We meet at a nearby restaurant, laughing, hugging. I haven't had a drink in four days. We order cocktail after cocktail, and by the time I leave to walk back downtown, I've drunk sixteen. And somehow, somewhere, between sixteen French martinis and a pitch-black stairwell, I fall down while walking upstairs. Plunging in the darkness, flying, until I hit a wall hard with my body at the bottom.

I crawl back upstairs on my hands and knees, and the next morning I wake with a screaming, sticky hangover and what later turns out to be a broken shoulder. I tell everyone how I fell in the darkness. How unsafe it was. How the hurricane has a lot to answer for. How it isn't my fault.

Six weeks later, it's Christmas in New York. The festivities, for me, have begun in earnest. One morning, a note on yellow paper is pushed under my door: 'Can you let me know you're OK? I'm really worried about you. Your neighbour, x'. Clutching it, cold fear takes hold of me. I search, scrape my brain, my empty memory, for the source of the concern. Last night was the work holiday party in an ornate, gilded-gold hotel bar with the colleagues I hate smiling for, smiling at every day. I ordered the strongest drinks they had, over and over, refusing the trays of tiny white food as my stomach spun and cramped and my chest tightened and I heaved.

There's a door number on the note. I fight the instinct to shrink and hide, dreading the knock on the door more than what I choose to do: walk downstairs and knock.

Knock, knock.

'Hi, I live upstairs. I got your note!'

'Oh God, are you OK?'

'I'm fine. Totally fine. Why would you ask?'

She starts to talk. She arrived home late last night, looked up the stairs as she jammed her key inside the lock and saw a pile: a gold dress, red shoes and a woman who looked like me inside them, lying unconscious. Gathering the woman in her arms, she'd asked:

'This is where you live, right? Are you OK? Can I call someone?'

'I live in Camden,' the woman replied. 'I need to get home to Camden. Where am I? Can you get me a cab?'

She'd dragged the woman inside, put her to bed. I laugh at her, at this woman, at that woman.

Just two weeks after this: a note on my front door, in different handwriting, stuck there for the day that I'd lain inside, not moving.

'Clean up your fucking mess. Your neighbour.'

A trail of food I don't recall being unable to hold in my hands, from the front door on the street to my door. I laugh at her, at this woman.

Four weeks more after this: another resident holds the door open for me, his face hardening as I say thank you without meeting his eyes. He recognises my voice.

'You're the one who comes in singing and shouting and crying in the middle of the night,' he says with barely disguised anger.

'Am I?' I ask.

Am I? I laugh, at her, at this woman.

Three weeks later: I'm leaving for work and the glass in the front door is smashed, the splinters and shards spread out like a delicate spider's web, trying to reach me. I stop; I flinch. I'm not sure I didn't do it. Did I? A picture lurks inside me: my foot, the door, I'm crying, angry. But is it a memory? A dream? Something I just imagined? It's pulled further into the sea that's flooded my brain and now it's beyond reach and I don't know, I'll never know.

I spend more and more time in the shadows, less time bothering to look for her. I know she's lost, if not gone entirely. The thin, sharp sheets that belong to someone else scratch my skin as I tug them tighter around me. The shouting and clamour and heat and spit and stab of the city collect on my shoulders. The weight makes my spine, my head, bend like the boughs of the trees that cover me. The weight comforts me even as it kills me.

I sleep.

I drink.

I drink.

Hours one and two I still feel lighter. So free. So myself. Hours three, four and five: the load gets strapped on, heavier than before, heavier than yesterday, somehow. My back buckles and the load snakes around each shoulder and forces its way inside my throat as I choke. I feel, I fear, that I can't survive this. I will die doing this. And it's OK, because I deserve this. I belong in this. I belong here. I'm at home. I can feel the fur under my toes. I tuck them under me, lay my head and prepare to rest. Hours six and seven are when the relief, the darkness comes and I feel nothing.

CHAPTER 17

Squatting within the shadows in the darkest corners of the city, I start to cut myself again. I don't remember the pebbly path of consideration, the thoughts and questions that would count as such. Or is it simply that my hands just picked up the blade – naturally, easily – without conscious, never mind careful thought? What day was it when thought became action and I carved myself up again? Though it will have been night. Deep night, the exact midpoint between the sun sinking and rising again. Of that I'm sure.

Did I ever stop? Really? If not physically still hunched over, belly over hips, as I opened up my own body until it was bloody, was I still there in my mind? Each period of time without its existence was a brief respite for my skin. A chance to refill. Little more than a chance for my blood to collect and pool inside me, ready to spill out when the silver sharp edge returned.

It might have been a while – how long? – but starting again is like breathing, sleeping. I know where to start, where to pick up where I left off – where I always do

– high and hidden. The tops of my arms, close to my shoulders while still being covered. The tops, the insides of my thighs. As things become worse, my aim becomes less precise, falls lower, sinks with speed and bursts out into plain sight. I slash at the inside of my arms, my wrists, my hands; then my neck and, for the first time, my face. The high pitch of pain runs through my bones until they rattle. I can't keep it inside and, once the surface is broken, it spills around my edges.

I develop a toolkit of increasing variety, the biggest addition lent by the professional chef's knives in the kitchen of my sublet. The rack of blades, pinned to wire on the wall, are of different shapes, sizes and sharpness. My eye trips over them as I step inside, causing a surge in my heart. I gaze at the knives, smitten, hypnotised by the light streaming across, bouncing off the blades. I'm in love, or, at least, lust.

I'd used knives before: knives that weren't sharp, had been cheap many years before, could barely make it through the outer skin of a small brown onion. How could I expect them to break and butcher human skin, my skin? Hard pulls of the serrated blade across my arm produced little blood – as I released it, tiny specks, like ink falling from the end of a fountain pen appeared on my skin. Faster, harder pulls have little more success, as does sawing, like through French bread, dry and flaking out of the oven. Each knife is filed inside my mind, sitting neatly alongside the razors that have been there a while.

I began with disposable razors but by now I've discovered, somewhat gleefully, that a razor blade out of the plastic works better. A blatant truth in retrospect, but a discovery I only made after, in a fit of frustration at being unable to cut my own skin, I smashed the pink plastic razor in my hands between my palm and the hard porcelain sink. The exposed jagged plastic was pushed into my greedy skin, and in that moment I discovered how quick, deep and painless it was initially to cut with just the blade. The pain, of course, came seconds later, but the absence of agony in the moment just made it easier to cut and cut and cut, deeper each time.

Until that moment, grip closed around the chunks of plastic and snapped razors, I'd been ruled by the thought that I deserved it to be hard. An easy, quick, clean cut was a gift. A gift, a simple solution that I hadn't earned yet, that I didn't deserve. So, each time I pressed the mound of plastic and blade into my arm, my leg, my neck, struggling to judge the angle, the pressure and the strength needed to achieve the desired mutilation, I felt comfortable with the difficulty and indignity of the task at hand. Each place and push, scrape and cut, never revealed the damage until it was done, the pressure and weight released.

Sometimes the skin would be scraped pink and raw. Sometimes it bore a cut – thin, precise, light. At other times I achieved a gash, deep and jagged, pulsing blood. Every time it hurt. Sometimes it really hurt. It, I, felt raw, sore, taut. The width, depth, shape of the wound was never consistent, always a surprise. My body was marked with holes, cuts, skin gouged out and chucked in the bin along with red-streaked tissues or towels when the job was bigger than a flannel.

As I hacked, stabbed and jabbed at my skin, I felt comforted by the discomfort, the difficulty, how hard it was to harm myself. The awkwardness and failed attempts folding inside me as my skin split open. The mixture of success and disappointment blending with the blood and skin.

But the intoxicating high it produced eventually paled next to the satisfaction I found with just a razor blade. The first time I tried it, clean, out of the head of a razor, I was hit by the heavy-eyed swoon of a straight, thin cut that opened me up like a grape bursting wide, spitting out its seeds. The rush of blood spilling out, pulsating and gushing and flowing silently, cascading and coursing down my arms and later across my wrists and round the tops of my thighs. The cooling trickle became a cold wave, the perfect salve for the burning on me, in me. I was red hot: every one of my organs baking and broiling. The rage and shame that imploded inside me, filling my body and rising up to touch the skin, turning me pink, hot to the touch, to the taste.

The morning after is always the worst. The night is a black blur – the flashes, flinching at the only glint of light bouncing off the silver blade under the orange light. The skin on my neck damp with tears, sticky with wine, the building, growing, morphing pain trying to push its way out of my chest when it fails to escape through my mouth, my eyes and ears.

At those moments, I see the bone in my chest explode open, a line carved straight down my middle, my skin and bones falling half to the left and half to the right. I think of the girl I'd survived a car crash with fourteen years earlier while travelling – she'd been stuck with gauze from her throat to her belly button, the wound spitting and spurting underneath. I used to imagine what she looked like with the gauze lifted off, and now I see my head on her body.

I'm cut from chin to tummy, split open, right in half. The pain's got teeth and chews a line from the inside out, spitting strips of flesh as it charges through me. When my body breaks, the only way I can put it back together, stitch it piece by piece, is with my own knife or any one of the razors and blades that I hold in my hands.

There isn't a calmness when I try to carve myself whole again. I always begin in the eye of madness: knee-deep in despair, crying, heaving. After the first time that I place the blade against my skin, press and pull hard, everything gets quiet. My pulse slows. It throbs inside my skull. My breathing loses its rapid, dancing rhythm. My face becomes dry, my skin pulled tight with salt. I concentrate on what I'm doing. How much it hurts. How bad it feels. How good it feels. But I know it can feel better; it can feel worse. Each time it doesn't hurt enough, or I don't bleed enough, I cut more, harder, longer, deeper. Summoning more courage – and it feels like immense bravery – to hurt myself *properly*.

More often than not, I go too far. Blood flows faster than I can catch it, control it. The cut springs open with a width and depth I'm not prepared for. I stare into the valley inside and think I can see a place I can be happy. I fall asleep on a crashing crescendo of pure happiness. The endorphins released like noxious gas when silver blade pares skin, reveals pain. My limbs ache with the pain of being peeled with steel; the stinging, high-pitched and taut, runs all over my body. I sleep easier than I have in days, sometimes weeks.

When the sunlight stirs me hours later, I feel the pain before I've fully opened my eyes. Shame rises like morning-after vomit in my mouth. I can't believe I did this again. It's going to take weeks to heal. How do I hide it? I want to grab the arms of the clock and pull them back until it's yesterday again and my skin is uncut. Panic gives way to practicalities as I work out how to bury myself in secrets.

Covering my cuts, burying my wounds becomes harder and harder. Plasters became gauze and tape and bandages. I take to wearing bracelets for the first time in a decade. Rows and rows of cheap plastic bangles, often worn up to my elbows. Stacked metal bracelets rub the cuts even more raw and sore. I put on long sleeves as the sun bears down. Barely scabbed cuts rub against the velvet, the polyester, the cotton. Opening up my arms means it hurts to sit at a table, with hands on the wooden surface. Opening up my legs means it hurts to sit completely still on a plastic chair, a cushioned chair, a sofa. When things are really bad it hurts to walk, to swing my arm in step. Each movement forwards, each forward motion provokes a rub, the sting of an open wound against fabric, snatching the breath from my mouth. I pick out the lint sticking inside the open red smiles with tweezers, knowing the metal will hit blood and nerves at some point and it will be all part of the punishment that I've come to deserve.

Then there's the night it's just not enough. No punishment is enough. There's no way to put myself back together and I want to walk into oblivion, pulling everything in with me. I take the blade to my forearm, press harder than I have ever before, furious at my loneliness, my sadness, the cycle of my own pathetic misery. I let out a sob-strangled roar as I pull the razor across.

My skin falls open like a mango as it spoils. Blood spits and spurts. I pinch together the skin, trying to magically make it stick back together, trying to stop the red wave. I panic, not because I'm hurt more than I intended – though what *did* I intend? – but because I don't want to go to the emergency room. I don't want them to know what I have done, to have to wear that layer of shame on the outside. To bear the consequences of what happens when you turn up at hospital with cut arms and flowing blood on the outside, not the inside. Everything is held together by a thread. The whole house of cards comes tumbling down if anyone realises how sick I've become.

It stops bleeding eventually. I pack tissue inside the hole. I wear new gauze, which blood stains quickly. There's no clothing which can cover what I've been doing. I wear dresses with short sleeves. No one asks me what I've done, how I injured myself, not here in New York.

When I go home to the UK they ask, alarmed: *oh my God, what have you done?* I tell them I caught my arm on a nail, tore it open as I pulled away. It's the only story that seems vaguely believable. Though I'm pretty sure no one does, in fact, believe me.

July 2013: it's the holiday weekend – a long weekend, with two whole days off work. I'm relieved, giddy. I meet a friend in Julius, the oldest operating gay bar in New York. The drinks – cocktails, vodka, whiskey, wine – slide down smoothly. I feed a line of dollar notes into the jukebox, selecting songs by Amy Winehouse, The Supremes and The Shangri-Las, before resting my body against the brightly lit box which hums from the vibrations of the heartache, loss and pain in their voices.

I twirl the bottle of Vicodin that's been rolling around the bottom of my handbag between my fingers. The white pills bounce, ricochet off their orange plastic home like a pinball machine. A fellow editor at work has gifted me with the full bottle, telling me that they made her vomit, were too strong. Not me. I have a strong constitution. The first time I swallow one, the stress, worry

138

and thrum of anxiety dissolves and drips out of me. Happy isn't the word; it's woefully inadequate to describe the state of perfect bliss I descend into, sinking lower and lower into the floor. It is walking on clouds with hands floating wide; it is singing from an open window as the wind flows through; it is a heart-shuddering, soul-heightening joy that I can never truly describe. A room of wool and twine in which I sit, knowing that I can do anything, everything, all of it, whenever I want. No one can stop me. Ever.

Now I know what real, true happiness feels like, I have to ration it, obviously. I can't truly begin to cope with what will happen when this happiness ends, is taken from me. This night, however, I know I'm owed it.

As the records end, load and spin underneath my hip, I swallow two tablets, then reach in my bag for a final one, just to be sure, tossing it into the back of my mouth, where it hits my throat, stuttering on the way down. I follow it with two Xanax. Then, almost immediately: nothing.

The next day, I wake up. I can barely open my eyes and keep them open when I do. I'm lying across the bed in yesterday's dress, ankle socks, shoes, beehive askew, hair grips lodged in the skin in my back, bag still over my shoulder. When I do manage to fully open my eyes I can barely see out of them – I fumble and find my phone: it's 1.30 p.m. My screen is filled with missed calls. I'm meant to be going to Coney Island with a group of women I know. I text one. Tell her I overslept.

Had a big night. She says they are worried about me. About what I was doing, what I'd done. I want to cancel with every bone and breath in my body but I can't. The shame on top of whatever else I'm feeling would just be too much. We arrange to meet; we're going to get the train together.

I haul my body off the quilt, my stomach already up in my mouth. I throw up once, twice; there's no food in my mouth because there'd been none in my stomach (I can't remember when I last ate). The vomit tastes of whisky, ginger, lime, wine, beer and acid. I get in the shower, counting the new small black bruises on me: my thigh, my arm, the bump on my head. I get out of the shower, vomit once more. I put on a new dress, new ankle socks and my brogues. Comb my matted hair, backcomb again. Spray, pat, spray, tease, smooth. I vomit again. Harder, longer. Blood hitting, splattering the bowl.

I make it to the subway station and onto the train. As it rocks and rolls towards Coney Island, I clutch my stomach, which is cramping and whirling under my fingers, under my skin. My mouth waters – squirts hitting both sides of my throat after being expelled from the glands. Sweat creates a trim the length of my hairline. At each and every stop I consider getting off, running through the doors, convinced I'm about to vomit violently, terrified I'm about to faint.

A little girl and her dad sit directly opposite me. Her pigtails are pulled tight on each side, her face taut. They both stare at me; her hand finds his, nervously. She's captivated and horrified by my face and I can't stop picturing hers in my head as I place my hands over my eyes and all I can see is black throbbing around her, framed by fireworks.

Somehow I manage to hold it inside until Coney Island, where I push my way out of the train and to the nearest trash can, which is already, on this boiling hot day, brimming over with discarded hotdogs, burgers, ice creams, sodas, ketchup-smeared fries.

With a primal urge that overtakes me, I grab each side of the can, which is open like a flower reaching for the sun. Food squeezes between my palms and the metal as I grab for my life, my head rearing back just once, snapping my body in half as it flips forwards and I vomit loudly.

As I buck and spew there's cheering and applause, heckling, from the other subway passengers. When my mouth is empty and my body still, I straighten my back, wipe my face with the back of my hand, spit and spew running between my fingers and down the outside of my hands, collecting at the wrists.

Eat something, I'm told by my kind-of friends, who have looked on in horror. Good idea. I queue for a hotdog and a beer by the beach. The line is thirty-something people deep. They're in shorts and vests, hugging, laughing and shrieking. I cower in their shadows, sweat running into my hair, down the centre of my back, down both legs into the heels of my shoes. The blue horizon in front of me waves and wobbles. My head swims; my body rocks.

The beer, the hotdog, have barely passed through my mouth and down my throat before they bounce back up, on a fierce wave that has me running, retching, to the most private spot I can find – the other side of a concrete wall. I splatter a new pile of bread roll, sausage and yellow liquid as neatly as possible onto the ground. It's enough, for all of us: they barely put up a fight when I say I must leave, must go home. That I can't do this, can't be here any longer.

I get another subway back, take a handful of blue sleeping pills and sleep until Sunday night. And just like that, two days and almost three nights have been lost. When I wake again, turn on my phone, I see pictures of everyone celebrating the holidays: on rooftops, on beaches, cocktails and sparklers in hand. While I lay unconscious, alone, they were living lives of joy, of love. A life I say I don't want.

CHAPTER 18

'Do you know,' says a woman in my office with a raised eyebrow, 'that the ratio of women to men in New York is two to one?' It's the statistic I hear most often and though it's not true, it feels like it is.

The other women are toned and tight, with bodies they get up at five a.m. to perfect and punish. They're perfectly made-up, with hair that they pay to have blow-dried most mornings. There are facials and brow-taming and leg waxing and vagina plucking. They are perfectly smooth and hair-free and their shiny faces glow. This is what it is to be a woman in New York. This is what men want.

It's not even that I feel out of my depth – I can't even begin to paddle in their pool. My hair is too bright and too broken and snaps between my fingers. I don't rip my pubic hair out with hot wax. My white belly folds over like sandwich crusts when I sit; my arms are corned beef. I've got black tattoos on my hands, my arms, my back.

Even though I'm slashing and cutting and drinking

myself into ugliness, I join dating sites, scroll past the men who all look the same, say things like, 'Looking for a partner in crime for workout dates' and 'No to drinking, drugs. Must be fit and no drama. No psychos.'

It's not unusual to see women of extraordinary beauty holding hands with men who are ordinary, sweating. Every man in New York believes he deserves the most beautiful of women. That he's entitled to her. And that we're duty bound to beautify and preen and primp ourselves for them. Anything less than that is a failure on our part.

Saturday night. I'm meeting my friend in the White Horse Tavern in the West Village. I arrive early, order a beer and take a seat at the bar. A man wearing a gold band on his left hand tries to make small talk. I limit my answers to nodding and smiling, with one-word accompaniments. My lack of conversation bothers him, the fact that I'm not responding to his attention needles him. He shakes his head and looks at me, from my toes to my head.

'It's such a shame,' he says. 'Those tattoos.'

I put my hand over my arm.

'What?' I say.

'They're just . . . fucking disgusting. It's like putting a bumper sticker on a Ferrari. Do you ever look in the mirror? You've ruined yourself.'

I swallow hard.

'Can you leave me alone, please?' And as he turns his back to me, I burst into tears, which splash off the bar.

144

A mean streak courses through the men of Manhattan. It fuels them and fires them. They dress it up as honesty and demand you're grateful. There's the forty-one-year-old who I go on two dates with after coming to in a Brooklyn bar to discover his mouth on my face and his hand all the way up my dress. I didn't know who he was or how we'd ended up in that dark corner. When I stand up to leave and he stands too, I realise he towers over me by a foot. To cover up my shame, I agree to a date with him as I leave. We meet for dinner, and midway through my bratwurst he says, out of nowhere, with no prompting: 'The thing is, I have no interest in a relationship right now. And God, definitely not a serious one.' After dinner, we go for a walk in a nearby graveyard.

There's the twenty-five-year-old who lives near me in the Village ('Well, I technically live with my parents. My dad's a filmmaker and my mom's an author'); is a writer ('Well, I suppose I'm a bartender really, but I have a blog'); straight(ish) ('Well, there are just too many cute boys in the world to say no!'; and was open to a relationship ('Well, I suppose I would be if the right person comes along but I don't *do* relationships').

There is the now-sober heroin and crack cocaine addict who texts me hourly after our date, not apparently needing a response. There's the Anglophile I meet on a dancefloor at a Britpop night in Brooklyn. Beard, hair cut just above his eyebrows, plaid shirt, black skinny jeans, Converse. The Williamsburg Uniform of Mediocrity.

'Ugh,' says one of the women I'm with. 'That's

Justin.' She leans heavily on that last syllable, balancing it like a razor blade on the tip of her tongue. 'He's so fucking boring.' The only thing receiving more emphasis than the last two letters of his name was the next sentence, whispered conspiratorially. 'He has cats.'

'Oh,' I say.

'No, you don't get it. Like, loads of cats. Seven, or something. And there's something wrong with most of them.'

'What is it you do?' I shout across the dancefloor – or was it by the bar? – as he strokes the torn, wet label of the beer he is cupping, watching me swallow a shot that gets stuck in my throat as it follows its path to my stomach, where it will sit for a few hours before retracing its original steps. I can tell by the arch of his left eyebrow that the man with seven sick cats is not much of a drinker and probably doesn't much care for those who are. I take great pride in drinking another shot to prove that I won't be stopped by the judgement of some man I barely know.

At some point, the man with seven sick cats asks for my number. He texts me the next day, as I lie between unchanged sheets and vomit sits in the toilet bowl. We arrange to meet at the White Horse pub, the site of the Bumper Sticker Guy. Sober, out in the daylight, without the tones of Jarvis Cocker to pull us into each other's orbit, we're both skittish and awkward. It turns out the answer to my question on the dancefloor was: 'A photographer. Well, not, you know, for money. I work in a camera shop, but I *am* a photographer too.' I ask enough questions, demure in the face of his obvious talent, his confidence bubbling up inside his chest.

'God, we used to get magazines like yours in,' he says. 'I couldn't even bear to touch it.' He shakes his head, rolls his tongue around in his mouth like he's eaten something bad. Something he wishes he'd just spat out. I flinch, unprepared. 'How can you live with yourself, really? Doing that for a living? It's just so stupid and pointless.'

'What?'

'Well, I'm just saying.'

'Well, don't,' I snap. I eye the door and consider leaving until he starts to pull us back towards safer ground. He's talking about the club night we met at while I recalibrate.

'. . . and you were flirting so outrageously with Jim.'

'Sorry?' I jerk my head up. 'Who?'

He smiles, but his eyes are dark as he says, 'The DJ. He's married, you know. You were throwing yourself at him!'

His laugh has a steely edge. I look at him, bewildered. I barely remember the face of the man who I requested song after song from, desperate to trick my body and brain into believing I was home.

'We were all talking about it afterwards. How obvious it was that you just wanted to sleep with him.'

Fury burns my chest.

'Yeah, I'm leaving,' I say, as I, with as much dignity as I can muster, which isn't that much, walk out of the

147

pub. I stand, swallowing the hot, toxic air into my lungs, feeling further away from home and happiness than ever.

Of course, this isn't the last time I see him. He takes me to his apartment in Washington Heights. We get the subway all the way up to the George Washington Bridge and beyond. When we get off, his New York is not mine downtown. He turns the key in the door and the smell of cat piss is overwhelming. His apartment is largely empty. A kitchen with two handfuls of crockery, glasses and cutlery. Next to it, the lounge, which is just a sofa bed and an office chair pulled up to a high computer desk. There's no TV. In the bedroom, he has a bed, a few books. The walls are bare and white-ish. His cats roam the rooms; they're on chairs and beds and behind doors. He introduces each to me individually, using a funny, high voice to speak directly to them. One is deaf; two are blind. Or were two deaf and one blind? One has diabetes. As I lie, shrinking on his sheets, they slink and stalk towards me on the tips of their paws; sensing my repulsion, they come closer.

I only attract, am attracted to, men who are at best apathetic or at worst cruel and cold. Whose emotions remain far away from me, kept on ice for the woman who deserves it. The path to my heart was marked out by the boots of my dad – some of the men who walk it follow his lead, put their footsteps in his. They find permission in his grooves, the blueprint for how to treat me. And I lose my ability – if I ever had it – to tell pleasure and love from pain and hate. It all feels the same for me, the language recognisable under my finger-tips. I love it when they hurt me and the hurt feels like love.

There are those who regard me as inessential to their life; they can smell, from both close and afar, the poverty, the shame, the trauma that has stuck to me from child-hood. Women like me aren't girlfriend material, never mind wife material. I drink too much, speak too plainly, swear too loudly, wear too much flesh and store too much below it. If I'm very lucky, they want to fuck me.

And I don't want them to but need them to because the truth I can't yet speak to anyone I know — only strangers who are blank pages for my confession — is that, after being completely sure that I never wanted marriage or kids in my twenties, I am now consumed with thoughts of both. 'By the time you're twenty-eight, ninety-eight per cent of your eggs have died,' says another woman from my office, setting off a tsunami of panic in my chest. I've never been further away from finding someone to love, who I could love enough to join myself with in two ways of such profound permanence.

But it isn't just a lack of a willing man. I'm still plagued by the horrors of my past, by thoughts of my own parents' irresponsibility. The bone-deep fear that shakes my voice is this: that I'll be a terrible mum. That I'm so scarred and twisted by my childhood that I'll be unable to do anything but repeat it. And that I'll not just be a bumbling, fumbling, doing-their-best new mum. But a *bad* mum. That the moment I have the seed of a baby in my belly, the very foundation of who I am will change. That the evil will flood my veins, overwhelm my brain. My eyes will blacken, my heart will stop beating and I will become a monster.

Now, however, the desire for a baby overwhelms my fear. I start to blurt it out to strangers at parties, people I barely know at work. 'Just go and sleep with any guy and don't use protection,' says one. Another sends me a link to an article on egg freezing. One night in Harlem, a gay couple, friends of a friend, offer me $10,000 to give them my eggs. I say no, but not as quickly as I'd have imagined.

CHAPTER 19

Summer 2013, after more than a full year in the apartment filled with darkness, I hit my limit: I can't squat in the darkness any longer, my skin being stripped off like bark. I wipe the knives clean, pack my bags and find a new place on Craigslist. For the first time in eight years, I won't be living alone, but I will be living in a room in an apartment where all of the light is kept: a straight-from-the-movies loft in SoHo. The bathroom is white and black-tiled, with a traditional claw tub. The living room is about six times the size of my old apartment – there are comfy sofas, a dining table for ten and big windows. *This* is the New York I came for.

I arrange a viewing with the live-in landlady, whose body constantly twitches, never still. She offers me a drink, talks manically, spits on me, and I see, feel, know, she's like me. My major concern about finding a new apartment, about living with another person – that my drinking would be too visible, that the state in which I came home most nights would be too visible – dissolves within seconds. I relax with relief. Most people wouldn't, couldn't live like that. But it seems we're kindred spirits. She clearly could and would.

The pop of a cork and she pours wine like it's water; her words follow – quick and clipped, ricocheting around the room before you can fully catch them. I recognise her, like her immediately.

'So?' she asks.

'Yes,' I say. 'I'd love to live with you.' We clink our glasses in celebration. The kindling is stacked.

Soon, she will crackle and break and leak in front of my eyes. I won't be far behind her. She's high on Adderall and weed and booze and possibly some other kind of unidentified uppers, and her whirling body and spiralling mind serve to distract me from mine. I'm taking Xanax and sleeping pills. They balance out the diet pills given to me by a personal trainer I know, after being smuggled in from Mexico. I've decided to take control: of my body if not my mind. To take a different kind of axe to my skin, to the fat below it. Breakfast is coffee, strong and hot; lunch is a small polystyrene carton of watery, tasteless vending-machine noodles; dinner is martinis, by the large icy glass. I want to starve my body, make myself disappear into the steam that shoots out of the deepest part of the city. When the voice saying *stop, don't, I'm hungry* gets too loud, I take another diet pill. They buzz through me, speeding up my body and brain and mouth. Then I don't want to eat. I want to talk; I want to write; I want to walk up and down Broadway for hours, criss-crossing the perfect grid of streets and avenues that makes up Manhattan.

My intense mania is only matched by hers and it hurtles towards me as I laugh and duck, caught in its slipstream. I spend hours looking at the windows of the penthouse apartments across from ours that look like the places normal, nice, sane people live. I imagine – sometimes dream of – their lives, the love, the families that sit inside. The happiness they enjoy.

The landlady turns up in my room – a square twelve-by-ten-foot purpose-built unit next to the living room – most mornings at six a.m., rearranging the two other pieces of furniture over and over again while I stir. She opens my door at midnight and puts her dog in bed with me, under the covers, while I sleep. She cleans with bleach all night long, talking to herself as she works her way through the whole apartment.

But some days and nights are worse than others.

It's five a.m. on a Monday morning. My alarm is set for 6.15 a.m.

Boom, boom, boom, boom. Smash. Clatter. Crack.

The noise of chair legs crashing and wine stems breaking and voices and bodies bouncing off into each other. The *boom-tish-boom* from the stereo is rattling the apartment walls and floors.

I pull the pillow over my head as the door to my room bursts wide. As my eyes open, she's already beneath the covers, a hand trying to find my hip, maybe something else. There's a man next to her I don't recognise and she's saying, 'Yeah, yeah, the three of us,' as I pull my knees up to my chest and lock my body tight, as I know how.

'No, no!'

She stops.

'Come onnnn!'

'I have to get up in an hour – can you leave?'

Silence.

'What are you doing?!'

They pause, roll their eyes, laugh at my rejection as they walk back through the door they barrelled through just seconds before.

I pull the pillow back over my head. A few minutes later, her head pops through the crack, as she asks: 'How about just him?'

I say no once more.

A few weeks later I wake up and my weave is missing. It's a vital friend. I'd started backcombing my hair a couple of years before, but knew that to get the hair, the height, the protection, I needed more. More than I had. So I'd developed a towering construction of socks and pads and extensions. Each morning I backcombed and pinned and sprayed until my hair was at a perfect ninety-degree angle. The more I fractured, the harder the sadness fell – the harder *I* fell – the higher, the tighter my hair became. I felt seen and invisible at the same time – I craved, needed both equally.

But now it's missing.

It was there when I went to bed, on my side table,

and now it's gone. The landlady denies all knowledge of its whereabouts or the circumstances in which it went missing. I go to work with a flat, small, naked head. I feel vulnerable and like everyone now sees who I really am. Someone says how young I look. Someone else tells me I'm pretty now. I feel bereft. Exposed. Like now, somehow, they can see my cuts, congealed blood, the pills that rattle around in the empty space just below.

Less than a week later, I arrive home, to the room that's really a box, and there, proudly, defiantly, in the centre of my bed is my weave. I look down the hallway: there's no sign of the landlady. I look around for clues. And there under the bed is a pair of purple knickers I don't recognise, that aren't mine.

The hot madness inside our apartment in the sky continues to build. I wake up one morning with tiny red bites on my body. I scratch my body, the bones that have made an appearance. 'I think the apartment has bed bugs,' I say to the landlady.

She reacts furiously: 'You must have brought them in!'

I struggle to remember why I'm here. I feel like I'm serving time, but I'm not sure for what. I work as hard, harder, than I've ever done, but my job leaves me feeling exhausted, emptier still. The women I meet smile and slip their hands into mine, the corners of their mouths never moving to meet their ears. The conversation stops when I enter a room. Words are said quickly, with sharp edges that cut, when I'm out of rooms. The person I've come here to be remains further away than ever before. I used to be able to see the outline of her, just ahead, but she's long gone now and I walk alone.

I've lived with loneliness before. I was a lonely child, a lonely teenager, a lonely adult. I have spent the majority of my life alone, mute, hiding. It's so soft and quick off the tongue, so easy to claim, romantic, even. But it becomes clear in this city that I've never experienced true loneliness before, not the kind that you wear like a cloak of invisibility. Loneliness layered upon loneliness until you wonder if you are, in fact, not just invisible, but dead already. Your existence snuffed out, suffocated.

I walk down Eighth Avenue and I believe, right down to my toes, that I can't be seen by a single person around me. The end result of the disappearing act I started a few months before. Now I'm in the air. In the sewers. In the spit on the sidewalk. Everywhere but in my own body.

When I was a kid I thought that the world was watching me – that human existence was me, and everyone else was just watching me. That the world started the minute I walked into a room, and stopped the minute I walked out. That I could communicate with the world through the mirror. That when I spoke into it, they listened, they saw. Now I'm not sure if I'd ever existed. That me, Terri, my consciousness, is a figment of someone else's imagination – maybe my own, if that is even possible. I try to talk to strangers just to check I'm there, here.

'Hello?' I ask the woman in a trench coat hurrying down Broadway on a Saturday afternoon.

'Excuse me?' to the man jumping into the cab I've hailed.

Neither so much as flinch in my direction.

I feel my identity, my sense of being crumbling. *Who am I? Where am I? What am I? Am I?* Maybe company will bring me back to life. I crave it: the look of recognition, familiarity in another's eyes. The fingers attached to the man in the bodega graze mine when he hands me my change after I buy cigarettes one night. The hairs on my arms stand to attention as 350 volts flood through my body. It's the first time I've been touched in months. I miss it so much. I miss feeling something, *anything* so much.

The drinking, the pill-popping continues. One night after a party at a friend's apartment, I take a handful of sleeping pills, half a handful more than usual. I feel myself drifting off, on the warmest, softest wave, and as it laps at my eyelids I think *this may actually be it*. It's not the first time I've felt this in recent months, but it is the first time I've so joyfully welcomed it. The relief as I sink further and further into the thick blanket, the arms of someone I love. I'm woken a day later, when my friend stops by to check I'm OK, still breathing, when I don't respond to his messages.

The cycle goes on, the darkness chokes, even in this place in the sky, in the light. Eighteen months after I left London, I decide it's time to go home. If I don't, something bad, something *worse* is going to happen to me. And it won't feel like that when it comes; it will feel good, like something better. It will feel like sweet, sweet escape. I quit with no job, for the first time in my career. For the first time, I choose life.

CHAPTER 20

I'm home, back in London. Within days, he appears, seemingly out of nowhere. But from the first half-moment, the first apparition, I know he's been there all along, moving as I move, forever just out of my eyeline. He's the one who was meant to find me, who I was going to come together in the hands, under the eyes, of.

He has a partner. I know this without asking or without him telling. I find it strangely, shockingly irrelevant. My usual concrete moral core barely flinches at my transgression: the joining of our bodies, his mind folding into mine.

His partner has nothing to do with me and certainly nothing to do with me and him. This isn't a convenient psychological dodge, a flinching away from the light so I can stack my guilt and regret neatly in dark corners. This isn't a belief that he doesn't love her, not really, hasn't touched the softest bit of her thighs in years. My obsessive imagination doesn't think about those moments beneath their sheets, the fact that they share sheets. She never intrudes on my mind. Sometimes I try to see her, force myself to conjure her from wool and fingernails and hair. See her hand in his, the joining of warm, familiar skin.

I believe he probably does love her; in fact, I'm sure he does. Just as I'm sure that his hands still find her body, pull her close in the middle of the night with an ache of tenderness and stab of desire. It's irrelevant. We exist elsewhere, as something else. There's no name for it, no words that can adequately articulate what and who and how it is.

The first message arrives out of the blue, but with the feel of an old friend, one that belonged to another time, another you. We make an arrangement, the very first one: we're to meet in a pub with flowers tumbling around the front door. And as I wait for him, knees tightly clenched, jaw set, I know, even though I can't possibly know, that this man has stained me. It starts to spread, tendrils pushing outwards, probing the holes and spaces in me.

He walks into the pub. The familiarity in the wave of his sandy hair and the arch of his blue eyes makes me ache. The first thing I feel is a sense of shattering loss that pulls my kneecaps tighter still. The loss of myself, of who I am, had been. Never has so much altered in so few seconds. On either side of a blink sit the old and new versions of me, of my life. After a second blink, I'm cascading over the other side into an unknown that feels known. The details of that first meeting are

160

a blur: what we say, what we drink. *Do we laugh?* I'm steadfastly concentrating on keeping the loss to myself, but it's everywhere – splashed up the walls, walked into the carpet, soaking through the cushions. It seeps back in through my skin and what will become a cycle begins.

When I sit, I think of him. When I sleep, I dream of him. When I walk, he's in my stride, in the bend of my elbow as an arm swings. He's invaded my brain and I can't get him out. I don't want him out. He's a stranger whom I know every inch and crack and crease of. The familiarity hums in our DNA.

There are more meetings packed with heat and longing; more dreams, texts, emails scratched out in the agony of absence. I gladly offer up my jaw as the yoke is fitted around my neck. I feel so in love and so insane. So desperate and deranged. Every sound is loud, bouncing uncomfortably off my ear drums; every colour I see burns through to the back of my eyes, turning the sockets black. I read about a woman who has her tear ducts cauterised, scars forming over and closing the pinprick holes shut. I want to burn my own to keep all of him, the chaos and ecstasy, inside me.

What can we do? What can be done? We can't be together – he says he's unable, unwilling to leave his relationship – but the very thought of the alternative tiptoes around a spiral I fear. The madness, frenzy, builds and builds, and just as all seems so desperate and lost, I'm offered a job back in New York, the city I'd left just weeks before. A job that I couldn't have sketched in my wildest of dreams. And just as I knew that if I stayed in New York, worse would happen, I know now that if I stay in London, worse will happen. To him, to me, to us.

I have to leave. I know I'm doing the right thing, am utterly convinced I am, but everything about it feels wrong, feels desperately like I'm doing something that will never ever be undone again. The hand at my back continues to push me away.

We decide to spend the weekend together before I leave. On Friday night, we meet in a pub where we think no one knows us. I spend the blurry hours and days before imagining the moment he walks in, the shot of endorphins hurtling through me, the electric shock that runs up my spine, makes me arch my back and bare my neck; I rattle on the wooden stool.

Then, as if I've summoned him from my imagination by chanting his name over and over again, he's there. The air escapes from the room through the open door and then he's by me, on me, fingers in my hair, his mouth on mine, fitting exactly as I'd remembered but still couldn't believe it ever did. The room swims and spins; lights blur and whirl and settle somewhere around the lines that sit in the pouch of skin between his thumb and first finger. I push my lips, my tongue inside, need the taste of him to take me away, away, away.

The next night, I wait for him in a hotel room, put on my favourite black dress that I hope is his favourite too, smooth it down, look at myself in the mirror, still shocked by how different I feel, look. *Who is she? Where is she from?* He knocks on the door, comes inside with a kiss. I keep opening my eyes to see if he's still there, still real. I can't believe he's a person in my hands; I touch him, constantly, trying to make him stay whole. But as I fill out beside him, he's disappearing next to me, becoming a ghost.

Hours later, I wake up, the sun is yet to rise and he's straight as a board next to me. Barely moving. Staring straight ahead. Panic strains, floods the sheets. *He has to leave; he can't be here; he can't breathe; he can't handle this.* Daylight comes and the words are the same. *He has to leave.* I know he has to leave. I know that he can't stay but I can't speak to tell him this. I know if I open my mouth, I'll gag or scream or any of the things that my body feels compelled to do. The life I've been finally given, the life that should have been mine all along is being ripped out of my arms.

I can't breathe. I want to ask him to stay. I want to *beg* him to stay, on my knees, hands on his thighs, but I can't. Instead I dress, stand, back against the roll-top bath, fingers gripping. He tells me *he can't, he's sorry, he won't. He must go back to where he must be.* I grip harder and harder until my pink fingers go white. Staring at the carpet, the swirls start to dance as spots blur and bend, becoming a dancing, writhing mass of bodies and brains.

As he's speaking – sounds that are noises, but not words – I feel part of me splinter and float up to the ceiling. She watches both of us as the scene plays out.

She thinks I'm pathetic. The way I look at the floor, tears burning my eyes, the way I swallow and grip, try to drill my emotion into the ground so that it sinks into the concrete and escapes him. She watches as the shutters go up, keeping me safe from what is happening around me, from what will certainly kill me.

I don't look as he shuts the door behind him, nor do I move. I stop feeling anything at all and I'm grateful for the numbness. I want my insides to be scooped out with a cold, steel spoon and dropped down the drains for the rats to ravage. Minutes pass, maybe hours. I don't move. I'm scared if I do I'll start to feel again.

Eventually, the sun starts to dim and there's nothing else to do but move. One foot, one hand, stretches out in front of the rest of me. I'm incapable of moving my body in one smooth motion, a movement that I recognise. One step and I'm on my knees, towels in my fist and then in my mouth. I'm choking but that's better than crying, than begging, than screaming his name.

When I'm dry, I pack my overnight bag, refusing to look at myself in the mirror as I move around the room and bathroom. I walk out of the door, unable, unwilling to turn around and take one last look at the room where we spent one night, the sheets still tangled and balled.

I walk down the hall, walls guiding me. I get in the lift, just big enough for two, press the button for the ground floor. I get out and approach the desk.

'Hello,' I think I say. We have a conversation, though I can't remember the words that pass between us as I pay the bill. Just seconds later, I'm out on the Soho street staring at the sky, at the lives being lived behind each tiny window. I feel it. He's gone.

Two days later, I'm on a plane to New York. I cry the whole way. The next morning, I'm up at four a.m., my sleep taken, too. I walk the streets of the Lower East Side as club kids fall, laughing, into yellow cabs and bodega owners in thick hats and vests cut through the twine holding stacks of newspapers together. He's 3,000 miles away and I'm more stuck inside him than ever. And now, without him, I don't know who I am any more, what's left. I wish I'd never met him. I can't imagine my life without him. I can't believe I existed without him. What do I do now?

CHAPTER 21

I know that my only salvation lies where it always has: with work. With this job that I've spent my life dreaming of. The career that has saved me every time I've been sucked into the sticky depths. It's also a chance to right all the previous wrongs, to prove that the city didn't defeat me. And that I'm good enough, smart enough, that *I'm enough*. For something, for someone.

It's a job working with a big, talented, suspicious, hard-edged team. I stand before them, the Empire State Building stacked in between buildings out of the window to my left, to tell them how great it will all be, how great I will be, as they stare hard in my direction. I'm in the office twelve hours a day, then tapping, chest tight, from home, or a bar, for several hours more. I pour every bit of my brain and energy into it. This will save me. This is who I am.

I pray that the pressure and constant thrum of stress will take my mind away from him. That I'll find sanctuary in the strung-together seconds when I no longer carry him around. I wait for the smallest sign – an email, a message, a picture, a word – a hint that I've spread inside his life like he has mine, that he too is altered. I hunker down in the dark, under the covers, scrolling, looking, waiting.

I write the first of many letters that I never send. Full of longing, lust and utter, desperate sadness. I write each one on the same paper, in the same blue ink, tearing the pages off when I'm done, folding them four times until I can't see the words, in the hope that they won't touch me. When that doesn't work I put them inside a plastic bag and turn that over four times too.

I think that he loves me. I know that he loves me. Each day bleeds to night, gives way to day, and it happens over and over again and I don't know when I'll see him again.

I dream of the day he means nothing to me, means less, when every single waking moment isn't owned, claimed by him. He squats inside my chest and I hate him and love him and want to cough him up out of my mouth and spit him into the air but he won't budge. I imagine what he's doing every minute of every day. I dream of him at night; he stalks my dreams; some nights he tells me it's OK, others he tells me it'll never be OK and I wake up gripping the sheets in my tight fists and I hate him more than ever. I want to kill him.

Saturdays, I pace Sixth Avenue. I try to keep in a straight line by putting food in my mouth and my feet on concrete but my mind flies away, out of my reach, across the sea and land, like a watchful bird, as he lies with the one he's with. He says he loves her; she says it back. It's no longer irrelevant.

I'll resign, I'll come home, we can be together, I plead from across the sea.

No, he says. *You can't do that.*

I can't do that. No.

I carry him on my back, across my thighs, around my neck. The weight is suffocating me. I can't breathe.

Being back in the city, the plague of before is never far away. I've been broken afresh, and in the seconds I can't control my thoughts, I feel apart from myself in a whole new way. My mind sitting so far away from my body. The world moving around me as I stand perfectly still, without comprehension. The wound is fresh, the dampness of new blood feels known, dangerous. Once again, within weeks, I'm burying myself in booze. The familiar clink and slosh comfort me while it chokes me.

Then, one night, I almost get arrested. I've been somewhere in the city, drinking alone. I flag a yellow taxi, climb in, share my apartment's cross streets before my head is lolling against the back seat as we speed home. I'm woken by the cab driver knocking on the plastic partition, announcing we're there and I need to pay. I scrabble around in the bottom of my bag: nothing. I try again. My purse is empty and there's no card – just loose change in there. I start to panic.

'I don't have my card,' I say.

'You have to pay,' he replies.

'I'm sorry. I don't know where it is.'

He shakes his head. 'If you don't pay I'll call the police.'

I panic, the panic of a drunk immigrant who knows they can be deported just for being arrested.

'Please don't,' I say and start to cry.

He locks the doors and calls the police. Several minutes later, there's a flash of police lights and a firm knock on the window.

'Miss, why won't you pay the driver? We'll have to arrest you if you don't.'

I continue to cry, my hand searching through my bag as they start to radio it in. Suddenly, it's there at the end of my fingers: the card that I was too hammered to find the other fifteen times I'd looked. The police keep their eyes on me while I pay, laughing.

'Miss, are you drunk?' they ask.

'No, sorry, I'm just tired,' I say, continuing to laugh while heavily tipping the driver so he'll lay off. The police finally let me out and I try to not so obviously weave through the West Village as they look at my retreating back.

While at night I battle with myself in the shadows, I'm reconciled on the outside during the day: the magazine has never been better, everyone agrees. What a great success. I'm finally enough.

The gap between these two halves of me grows. I reach upwards, outwards, push harder, straining, as the crack beneath me widens. I exist in the gap and it's wonderful. I sit in absence, in complete isolation and

I'm made steady, almost completely frozen by the singularity of it. This, I can understand. Here, I think, I can be. Here, I am nothing real. I don't feel, and when I do, I stamp the last orangey embers out under my boot.

I go instead, most nights, to the place where you pay to feel for three minutes. I can't remember when and how it first seemed like a sensible avenue for treating my madness. It does, after all, go hand in hand with my drinking, like a pair of intimate sisters, fingers slipped into a warm, soft palm after the correct number of drinks (four, by the way).

My apartment in the East Village is just three blocks from a karaoke bar, which is itself another five or six from another karaoke bar and so on and so on. There are so many karaoke bars in New York that you could navigate the city by the bright, flashing, sticky neon squares of abandon that light your path alone.

My favourite bar, the one that I became a weekly, twice-weekly, thrice-weekly visitor to is on St Mark's, up brownstone steps and inside high-ceilinged rooms. On the odd occasion I manage to convince someone to come with me, but more often than not, I go alone.

The staff know me by now, pitying looks in their eyes. The sad, drunk girl back again. I always sing the same songs: 'You Oughta Know' by Alanis Morissette; 'It's All Coming Back To Me Now' by Celine Dion. Melodramatic songs of loss, regret, rage, betrayal. I always play the same trick: slipping the unamused bartender a twenty-dollar bill with each song request, barely registering that I was dropping, in total, about a hundred bucks per night. Or that it really seemed to make no difference to when my song was played. Still, I folded the bill in four, slipped it into her hand underneath the song slip I'd filled out, clutching her hand for a moment as I pressed it in with a smile and a raised, knowing eyebrow.

I always drink the same drinks: a beer and a Big Apple (an apple martini in a plastic glass with a few cubes of sticky ice). I sit at the bar, waiting for my turn. When I'm up, I leap to my feet, clasp the microphone with both hands like my life depends on it, which it basically does. Sometimes I pull the air into me through my fists; at others I bend my knees, before my body lurches back upwards; on the worst nights I fall to my knees, head bowed towards the concrete floor as I pray and sing.

I never remember leaving. I wake up after each karaoke night at home. I can't tell you if I'd walked the blocks or got a cab. I can't tell you when or why I ordered food when I got home – curry, burgers, chicken, a cheese toastie – the detritus in the morning sometimes in a pile on the couch, sometimes stuck to my thighs, sometimes under my head and squashed into the pillow, sometimes scattered across the sheets like wedding-night confetti falling out of underclothes.

The next night, four drinks in, I walk through the door at the top of the stairs, the heads of the staff who pour the drinks and cue up the songs jerking back, recoiling in recognition. And it begins again.

I imagine that I'll find solace in the space between the songs and the sadness and the drinking. I'll find myself, crouching from view. I think that the songs are a path to the emotions I can no longer access naturally, only through the spit and shriek of public singing. In those moments, I feel full; I feel love, hate, fear, lust, anger. The feelings building, swelling and shrinking as the music moves. When it ends, fades away, the emotions leave me, leave my body, and I stand as empty and cold as the moments before it began.

The darkness is back, in full song, draining colour and life from everything.

CHAPTER 22

Karaoke was a doomed saviour, but one I sought out, because my condition was worst in the evenings. As the sun set, hope swirled away to be replaced by deep, cellular fear, my entire body erect and alert. Growing in dark corners, like the night-blooming cereus, waiting for the moon to peel open her petals and welcome life in. But I'm not welcoming life in. I'm welcoming the absence of it. I know every night I lie spread wide: everything is at stake again. Will I make it to the other side? To the rising of the light again? Will I be happy that I have?

Trying to place my arms, even my hands, around the fear is not just difficult – it's impossible. It's a totality I can't comprehend. But I can see and identify and speak to shapes, fragments of the fear.

The fear is this: that I'll never live happily and quietly, only violently and in pain.

The fear is this: that I'll never love, truly, never be loved, truly.

The fear is this: that I'll never be stitched together;

my secrets, my indignities, my humiliations, my violations, my shame will flap, slap noisily against the loose bones that rub my skin red, rub my skin raw.

The fear is this: that the fog will snake and choke, trapping my breath. That I won't wake, won't stand and put my left foot upon the floor. That the moment will have swallowed me whole, swallowed me alive.

The fear is this: that the fog won't snake and choke but choose to let me breathe. That I'll wake, that I'll stand and put my left foot upon the floor. That the moment will pass, as it always does, before blooming in my belly, curdling as it swells.

Every morning sees the beginnings of hope, the promise of growth, and then every night it turns inwards and withers all over again. Once the taste of death has been under your tongue, lodged along the edges of your gums, it never leaves your mouth. Ever. It's not always the first thing you smack your lips at when you wake up or the last thing you savour before your senses shut down for the night. But you can hack and rinse and spit as much as you like – it always remains and it takes little to bring the taste vividly into the present. The sight of the sea through a window. The sound of waves crashing against rocks. A butter knife glinting in the sunlight that hits the cutlery drawer as you open it.

I sleep very little, just lie unconscious for a few hours, so spend hours in the dawn light imagining the various ways, the minute intricacies of the methods on offer. The fantasies set my pulse racing, my heart skipping: I stick a pair of scissors in my neck, mouth pulled tight, silently screaming at the cracks in the ceiling; with all my strength, I pull the blade of the knife down, across and around my throat in a circular motion as the blood shoots out and the fatty skin swells and contracts. I feel the thick rope between my fingers, see my body standing on the bed to loop the rope around the light fitting, feeling the rub against my neck as I place my head within its jaws. I taste the pills as they speed over my tongue into the back of my throat, falling down into my belly. I stand on top of the cliff, wind whipping my hair, and close my eyes as I jump: first my right leg and then the left trailing a little behind. They flail and whirl as I fall fast, my body breaking into pieces as it hits the concrete water. I steal a red pick-up truck, loop a pipe from the exhaust, wind the windows up tight, turn on the radio and sit and wait, breathing in the end.

I read about a young woman who threw herself off the George Washington Bridge, leaving her Xanax and her handbag behind. I follow in her path. Step into the footprints she left behind her retreating frame, across the brow of the bridge to the spot that she'd chosen to jump to her death.

It becomes an obsession that coils around the insides of my mind, tainting everything it touches until my brain is flooded by thoughts of suicide. There is no room for any other thoughts, any other dreams.

I find a website that lists all methods of suicide, rating them for pain and statistical likelihood of success. I rank my preferred methods, praying for the intersection of little pain and high chances of success. It tells me that for each one successful suicide attempt, there are thirty-three unsuccessful ones. It assures me that 'for anyone committed to killing themselves, achieving the goal can be straightforward if a reliable method is chosen'. This makes me feel comforted; it makes me feel rational. I'm applying logic to my decision.

There is, as it turns out, no painless way to die. I measure the presumed physical pain against the mental pain I am currently collapsing inwards under. If the latter is unbearable, would the former be bearable because it would mean the end of what I couldn't take? And how much does it hurt? How much pain is there in a bullet speeding into your brain, your heart? What do you know, feel, before you know and feel nothing? If hanging doesn't break your neck, and you die by suffocation, how much pain is there and for how long?

I've written five, maybe six suicide notes in my life. It strikes me as something you should probably remember: the specific number of times you've put your final message to the world on paper, in ink, in pencil, in last-resort lipstick, the precise set of circumstances around each one. To give it the gravity, the weight it's supposed to hold, if nothing else. The smooth barrel of the pen between my second and third finger; the faint blue lines marking out the path my words are to travel; the bone in my right wrist scuffing the paper as they creep across in single file.

But that's not how it works. It's snatches, shapes, sounds, fragments, shadows, small sharp stories of despair and, at the very middle of me, of it, five or six notes saying: *I'm sorry. I can't. I won't.* And, now that I think on it, it may well even be seven. Not that it matters especially, even if it should.

The time I will come closest to succeeding and dying, I won't actually write a note at all. Not a word. Not a second in which I pause with a pen or scarlet lipstick tube ready to load and fire. For there will be no thought at all, only doing, doing, doing, until it is done. Well, almost done. Almost.

The reality is that if I had the presence of mind, the gathering of mind, to write a note, or the time to herald my thoughts into a linear enough line to begin to produce one, then that, right there, was an opportunity for doubt to invade, ants marching in a line through the cracks. Once inside, they make a home, thatch and nest, sprout wings out of the line in their backs and duplicate over and over until you can't see, feel, the cracks of my mind. They're obliterated by a marching, bobbing crater of bouncing black, the doubt made fear.

Each time I failed – I survived, I lived – it was the fear that was to blame. Not the fear of death, of not existing: I feared the living experience of trying to die, of the process of suicide. The fear that it would work, kind of, but not quite well enough. I'd be left trapped inside the shell of my still-functioning body, unable to speak or move or talk or walk but just conscious enough.

That I'd be myself, just physically broken, stuck back together with tape, never to get better.

The fear of causing my family pain. I could feel their sadness, touch their anger: the questions I'd never be able to answer, the guilt they didn't deserve, hadn't earned.

I knew how it would look. I knew what others would say. I knew how my obituary would read. They'd ask why, ask how they didn't know, how I hid it. I was furious. How could they claim not to know? Could they not hear me? Could they not see me? I've always, always known that there is an exit, a door, just off to the left of me where others couldn't see it. I like it. Knowing it is there, an option, if it ever feels like I have to step off, step out. My fingers brush against the door jamb, the edges, fingertips cooled by the draught that sat in the gap.

Each time I failed, I'd be ashamed that I hadn't been strong enough, that I'd allowed fear to win. Why wasn't I strong enough? Determined enough? Resilient to the pain, unflinching under its heat. Lying, spreadeagled, straight and stiff, jaw locked, teeth tight as the life was sucked out of me. Resistance giving way to relief.

It's hard to live when you suspect your life ended at five. But was that even possible if I wasn't even a fully fledged person by then? The years from then have been spent trying to give myself reasons to live. To say to myself: your life is worth something. You're worth something. You're worth trying to save over and over again.

I will save you every time you need it. I will save you until you're able to save yourself.

The hours of fantasy about how I will die are followed by hours of shame. Shame for what is filling my brain until it feels as though it will burst and shatter. My shame tells me that maybe I should get help, while my brain tells me that I should just get on with it. I realise that all I really know for sure is that this, this daily existence, even with the fantasies, has become unbearable. The pain of limbo – of living a life which is wholly concerned with death – is bending me in half every day.

I let my shame take the lead. I run my insurance details and 'problem' through a website that gives me a short – very short – list of doctors whom I can see. However, if I'm willing to go outside my insurance and pay, I can see almost three times as many doctors. Each one describes a specialism: PTSD, eating disorders, sexual trauma, self-harm, addiction issues. I try to rank my problems in order of importance. The most pressing one + my insurance + a doctor on the island of Manhattan = the answer.

I end up choosing by the next available appointment, convinced if I have to wait a week, I won't make it. The next day, I have an appointment with a fifty-something male doctor on the Upper East Side. I step out of the elevator onto the floor of his office, where a thin-lipped secretary sits tucked tight into the corner. Her job seems to be equal parts charging your credit card and welcoming you to the office. A brown and beige office on the outside and inside. I sit on a chair against the wall, one of just two, waiting to be called through the door that's touching my left shoulder. I run through what I should say in my head. *How much of the truth should I tell? Do I tell him how I feel right now? Or how I've felt my entire life? Where do I begin? Where would I even end?*

I'm called inside his airless office. It's tiny and tight, little to no light streaming through the blinds that cover both windows. One is almost entirely obscured by the churning, chugging AC unit, covered in dust, spitting out lukewarm air. The other looks out onto another brick building. He looks at me through his wide glasses, weary but ready to hear what I have to say. The words that come out of my mouth are jumbled, jangling. Later I struggle to remember exactly what I told him in my five-or-so-minute speech but I think I talk about my drinking, my shame, my pain, my abuse, my self-harm, my bloodied arms and black insides, how everything goes bad, goes wrong. I think I cry.

He nods, writing down as I speak. He pauses when I eventually stop, spent, and says, 'It sounds to me like you have borderline personality disorder.' He says that my trauma wired my brain differently. He prescribes mood stabilisers and anti-depressants. I forget to ask any questions, take my prescriptions from his hands and I'm back in the hall, confused and relieved. Relieved that after all these years, I have a name for what's wrong with me. I have pills that will make it better. Maybe they'll even make me not want to die, I think. Or feel a little bit more like living.

I google as soon as I've offered up my credit card, been dispatched in the lift and am back out on the street. There are generally accepted to be nine symptoms of borderline personality disorder:

1) Fear of abandonment
2) Unstable relationships
3) Unclear or unstable self-image
4) Impulsive, self-destructive behaviours
5) Self-harm
6) Extreme emotional mood swings
7) Chronic feelings of emptiness
8) Explosive anger
9) Feeling suspicious or out of touch with reality

I think of the blades I've snapped out of my plastic razors and taken to my skin. I think of the moments – too many to count – when I've felt hollowed out, as if at my very core there is nothing but air and space. I think of the rage that makes my vision blur. I think of the heart-stopping desperation when I'm left or in fear of being left. I think of the minutes when the feelings and emotions I can't separate out reverberate off the walls.

I go to the pharmacy a couple of blocks away to get my prescriptions. Two orange bottles containing my hope. I take them home and put them on the white bedside table unopened. I choose not to take one that day. I don't ask why. The next day, the same. By the third day I know that I'm saving them. Two full pill bottles could be the answer to a different question. Knowing they're there makes me feel safe, makes me feel that it'll all be OK. They're the way out when the time comes. And I know, instinctively, that the time is coming.

CHAPTER 23

At the same time that my mind is breaking, my body begins to buckle. I stop eating. I lose half a stone, finally arriving at the weight I've always wanted to be. My legs spasm. My brain feels like cotton wool. My skull fuzzes from the inside as what feels like volts of electricity run between the left ear and the right. I have pins and needles in my hands, my feet. I fall over in the street. I feel anxious and absent and out of sorts. Something is wrong, I know it. I'm coming undone, bone by bone, muscle by muscle, organ by organ, cell by cell.

The doctor bangs a small hammer against my knees and elbows, shines a light in my eyes, asks me to grip her arm, hard. Due to the luck of my insurance, I'm sent for an MRI the next day. I tell the doctor that I'm claustrophobic, can't breathe in small spaces, won't be able to spend what I'm told will be forty-five minutes lying in a tube in a machine. She reassures me that they'll give me Valium and ensure I'm comfortable. I arrive at the imaging centre, referral in hand. The woman behind the desk takes it brusquely from me.

'When will I take the Valium?' I ask.

'What?' she snaps. 'No. There needs to be a specific doctor here to administer that and he's only here on Tuesdays. If you want your scan today, you need to do it without.'

I nod, embarrassed, hand to my throat as it tightens. After waiting a while, I'm taken downstairs and given a gown to change into and a locker to place my clothes and shoes in. I sit, holding the gown around me, wishing I'd brought socks for my bare feet which are trailing on the cold floor. I'm taken through to the room with the MRI machine, the technician comes in, tells me that it'll last about forty-five minutes, that the noises the machine makes may be loud and disorientating but I need to lie completely still so that the scans, the pictures, are taken properly, can be read. I lie down. My head is strapped in place, I'm given earplugs and closed in on both sides. The technician leaves the room and his voice comes over the speakers:

'We're going to start the machine now and you'll move inside.'

The surface I'm lying on slides inside the scanner slowly, and my breath quickens, trebles in speed.

'Now you'll hear some loud noises.'

A throbbing, clanking, banging noise starts pulsating through the machine and vibrating into my body, shaking my eyeballs loose.

I try to keep calm but the roof of the tube I'm inside is just a couple of inches away from my face. I'm being buried alive, trapped, I can't move my body; my breath hits the ceiling and bounces right back down at me. The noise is so loud I feel like I'm consumed by it.

It's the sound of a workman's drill meets a round of live ammo, mixed with European house music that you can only hear at five a.m. when your brain is scrambled and your pupils full. *Just one more second*, I tell myself repeatedly. I don't work out how many seconds there are in forty-five minutes. Although the scan is done in three parts and they offer to let me out between each section, I say no: I want this over as soon as possible. The tears pool under my static head.

The next day, I receive a call from the doctor's office, calling me in. She tells me that not all of my scans came out entirely clearly but that they can see what look like lesions on my brain. The world stops entirely for a moment, just a millisecond before it bounces and catches up with itself, carrying on as it did before, leaving me behind this time. I'm googling as she speaks. The results: multiple sclerosis.

She tells me not to panic, that she's going to refer me to the MS specialist centre, but that there are other things that can cause these lesions: Lyme disease, Parkinson's and other autoimmune disorders. But none, nothing at that moment, seems as bad as MS. As losing my ability to walk, to swallow, to care for myself. I'm alone in the world: how does someone who has no one to care for them survive this? My appointment's a week away – at one of the best centres in the world – and I spend the week googling feverishly, looking for stories of successful recovery. I drink even more than I do usually and panic three times daily that the Xanax isn't in the bottom of my bag at all times.

I go to the centre with my friend. I'm given the same examination by a new doctor – a hammer to the knees and elbows, a grip and a grab – and she asks me to join her at the desk. She says, 'Look, there's nothing conclusive in your scan: some of them are blurred; there are lesions, but who knows what they're from. The only way to diagnose if it is MS – and there's no indication currently that it is – is to see you over a period of time, so we'll monitor you and do a follow-up scan.'

The relief rolls off my shoulders. I feel liberated and free, like I've been given my life back. A few months later, I'm given another scan. The doctor leaves a voicemail. I call her back. Nothing necessarily to worry about, she says, but there's something behind my eye they'd like to take a look at. She asks me to go back in. I delete the message; I never go back.

A week later, I overdose.

CHAPTER 24

D ay One in the psych ward. 5.30 a.m. Low, steady voices wake me. I haven't actually been asleep that long, having woken in panic every time the night staff did their bed checks, every ten minutes.

One of the voices I hear now has a thick, sharp accent. I open my eyes, trying to work out where I am and who's speaking. The voice sounds foreign, definitely non-American, possibly European. My eyes begin to focus on the wall I'm facing; through the mesh I see the city, made from shadows and false light, under the still-dark sky outside. I take a breath and turn over to see to whom the voices belong. There's an elderly woman with white tightly cropped hair sitting in the bed next to me, the bed that was empty when I fell asleep. She's being washed by a nurse, her nightgown pulled down. Her breasts, lined, wrinkled and brown, rest on the white sheets. She offers up an arm to be washed, and then the other, the white hairs on her arm standing up for inspection under the yellow strip-light over her bed.

I watch out of half-closed eyes. I don't want either of them to see me watching. I don't want to talk, make polite conversation with a new, mad, topless woman. I've only been here a handful of hours and still can't believe this is now my reality. I shut my eyes tighter, desperate to make them go away, but the hum and the hard consonants crash into my peace. I turn back over, pull the blanket up to my chin and will myself to sleep, the only place I can escape and be free from the insanity all around me.

A couple of hours later and I'm awake again. The woman next to me is sitting up in bed, reading, her nightie pulled up now, her breasts safely encased inside her bra. She peers at me over the edge of her reading glasses as if she's only just noticed me. She's in her seventies, has a strong, chiselled jaw, pronounced eye sockets, strong, arched nose, nostrils like almonds. She's tanned, speckled and sprinkled with brown marks that the sun has given her body. I'll soon see that she walks with a slight stoop, her legs swollen and coarse, a layer of softness over her thighs and stomach that dances when she walks, swaying slightly side to side.

'Hello,' she says, offering her handshake, overjoyed to hear that I'm also a foreigner when I reply. She's an artist, she's called Ana. She splits her time between San Francisco, New York and Berlin. She eyes me carefully. 'Are you a reader?' *Yes, yes I am.* She seems happy. 'Oh, thank heavens I'm sharing with you,' she says, and then: 'Ugh, I bet everyone in here is crazy.' I laugh, feel a momentary lightness as I do. Buoyed by her recognition – *I'm* not like them. I'm like her. Normal.

She doesn't want to come with me to breakfast, but I feel I must go. It's what sane people do and I'm conscious of the Note Takers. I put on the hospital gown, the socks, my hair, the bits of make-up I've been allowed to keep. I look in the mirror above the sink in the bathroom and try to work out if I could smash it and use the pieces against, on, myself. I could smash it with a chair, with my fist, with my head. How much could I pull out and use in the right place before they came in and here and got me? Not enough, I think. Not enough.

I take a deep breath, walk out into the hallway, join the steady stream of people moving towards the corridor where the food trolleys are parked. I hold the back of my gown together, try to keep the heat out of my cheeks as the other patients look at my New Girl Gown and Just Admitted Socks.

'Hi,' says a nurse. 'Terri? As you weren't here in time to order your breakfast, you'll just have to take what's left over.'

I wait until all the other patients have taken their trays – their names called out one by one, surnames only – and have cereal, milk and juice. Taking my tray, I walk into the dining room (cum therapy room, cum meeting room) and look around nervously. Small groups sit together, nothing outwardly noticeable binding them into their gangs. They look up as I shuffle into the room in my socks, then look at each other. No one makes eye contact with me, to let me know it's OK, they get it; they've been here too. But then I spot a woman on her own. Brown hair, unbrushed and knotted like rope, that keeps falling in her eyes as she blinks it away, never moving it away, out, with her fingers. The dark circles swallow her eyes, her T-shirt is stained and her soft belly rests over the waistband of her jogging bottoms. I walk over to the table.

'Hello, how are you?'

She stares.

'I'm Terri,' I say by way of an introduction that she definitely didn't ask for.

'Would I be able to sit down?'

She doesn't respond. I nod at the chairs.

'Can I?'

She looks away. I take this as a yes and sit down, the whole room going back to their conversations once I open my carton of milk. She never looks up again, pushing her spoon into her mouth before she's finished swallowing what was last put in there.

After breakfast, we form another line (there is a *lot* of queueing in psych wards). We have our temperature, pulse and blood pressure taken, one by one, sitting in the plastic chair opposite the nurses' station. We then queue up again to get our meds. Once you hit the front, the nurse checks your wristband and your medical forms and gives you your medication in a small paper cup. Just like in the movies. You have to swallow them as they watch, stick your tongue out in proof. Just like in the movies. I've been prescribed Prozac and propranolol. I will tell the doctor that I feel better immediately. I don't. I don't feel anything. Not a single tremor or tickle. But I need him to believe in my transformation: the epiphany of medication, the pharmaceutical salvation that he's charged in with, clasping it in his hand like an unsheathed sword.

I panic at how I'm coming across. I know that I can seem cold, hard. Judgemental and superior, even. And at times, I am all of these things and worse. I'm trembling with nerves and fear, the twisting and spinning of my guts. But I need to make sure none of this spills out. If I let my brain and body go, they'll never be reconciled again.

I've read those awful stories in the paper: those people who threw themselves under trains, surviving while the train kept them together, falling to bits as the car is lifted off them. But the cuts, the incisions which severed, chopped me up, couldn't be seen to the naked eye. So, for now, all of my effort has to be spent ensuring that it stays this way. Falling apart here and getting fixed isn't even an option. I can't allow that to happen. I won't.

Later that morning, I meet with the doctor. It's Friday. I realise this is the last chance to get out before the weekend. In my notebook I've written, in pencil, 'WHAT'S THE PLAN?' The conversation goes like this:

'So, how are you feeling?'

'Oh my God, so much better!'

'Really?'

'Oh God, yes! I think I was just stressed and drinking too much and I feel so much better already! What a wake-up call! I'm so grateful for this experience!'

The doctor nods, doesn't talk and writes. 'There's an AA meeting in the hospital tomorrow. It's not arranged by the hospital, we just allow them to host meetings here. I think it could benefit you to go.' A pause. 'What do you think?'

'Um, sure,' I say. 'If I'm still here. But what I really wanted to talk about was going home.'

The doctor shakes his head. 'Nope, you won't be going home before the weekend.'

I swallow hard.

'Well, Sunday is day three. And I was originally told that I'd be here three days. So, can I go home then?'

'No,' he says. 'Doctors aren't here on the weekends – no one's discharged then.'

'Monday?' I counter, eyebrows raised, face strained, ready to flinch at the next rejection. I can feel my escape slipping further through my hands, an eel wriggling and slipping through the gaps between my fingers; I can't hold on to it.

'You need to concentrate on working on yourself, on *really* getting better,' he says. I don't know what he means. Aren't I already better?

It's explained to me, very slowly, in very specific terms by the doctor, that it'll go in my favour if I participate in the entirely voluntary group sessions. The piece of paper on the wall breaks down exactly what and when they are, along with the allotted times for breakfast, TV, lunch, telephone calls, dinner. Each segment is witnessed and marshalled by a member of the ward staff. They stand off to the side taking constant notes. I wonder of what. Whether we're joining in? Looking happy? I spend my time joining every group going, convinced that this is my way out, smile slapped across my face. The nurses, attendants, stand and they write and write and write. They look at their watches, look at all of us, write and write some more. Pages and pages. They're constantly observing. I long to spend all my time in my room lying down but I know the isolation will go against me. That it's a sign of depression, of not committing to treatment.

So, I decide: I will wake every morning in plenty of time for breakfast, a meal that I've never eaten. I will shower. I will do my make-up. It's important that they can see me taking part in my usual rituals, not that they know what my usual rituals are. I'll smear the foundation over my face. When it's completely covered, I will paint on my other features: the liquid eyeliner, while being careful not to have a shaky line (I imagine the notes – *This morning, Terri had wobbly eyeliner. She looked full nuts. Keep her in another month. No, two!*). Instead, a thick, steady line from the corner of my inner eyelid to middle, pause, lift off the liner, place it back on exactly where I stopped and draw to the exact point my eye stops. I will then find a point, at an angle, two inches away, draw a dot and join the lines, before colouring in the thick lines.

193

Then I'll brush each lash of each eye, top and bottom, with black mascara. My lipstick, red, will be painted on – first the outline of my mouth, then I'll colour in until it's a red mass of flesh in the middle of the white. I'll practise smiling. Does it look more natural if I show my teeth or keep my mouth closed? (New note: *Terri was smiling like the Joker when she took her breakfast tray. Must be mad. Another two weeks! Hell, three to be safe.*)

The final part of my daily ritual – when I'll attach my hair, erect, fat, sticky.

I can't work out if this will be putting myself back together each day or simply painting the façade afresh, like the houses on the island of Mykonos that are painted every year to cover the damage from the sun and the sea whipping off the white and showing the brown layers underneath.

Whether I'm continuing the sideshow, and what that sideshow is and why I'm performing it is, I decide, not ultimately what really matters. The priority is getting the hell out of here as quickly as I possibly can, and if that means painting myself up like a clown, I'm all for it.

My performance can begin.

CHAPTER 25

The next morning. Seven a.m. Ana is already awake when I open my eyes. She's smearing make-up up, down, under and over her face. Following the curves and contours of the front and sides of her skull. I ask how she is, invite her to come to breakfast with me.

'Aaagh, I can't,' she says. 'This place . . . crazy people drive me insane.'

I smile. 'Yeah, I know what you mean.'

'You are not mad,' she says, matter-of-fact. 'Why are you here?'

I tell her about the drinking, the pills, the overdose – the slippery path that saw me stumble until I fell down this particular hole. How I don't know how to get myself out. She's nodding. 'You're a perfectly sane person who just loves to drink!' she says, both reassuring and offending me. 'Like me,' she continues brightly and then tells me her story. After several weeks of insomnia – and three straight days awake – she'd brought herself to the ER, desperate to get something to help her sleep. Somehow, between admitting that she drank several glasses of wine every day and battled crippling, crushing insomnia, that she hadn't slept for seventy-two hours, she'd been told she couldn't now go home – to any one of her homes, including her 'very large' apartment on the Upper West Side.

'Did you sign some forms?' I ask.

'Maybe . . . I don't know!' she says. 'I was just so tired and wanted to sleep. But now they won't let me out. They say I'd have to appeal. I'll just do my three days.'

'But what if they won't let you out after that?' I say, articulating my deep fear. I am really testing the water for my own path forwards. Trying to work out the likelihood that I won't be able to get out. Aware that my own day three is tomorrow.

She shrugs. 'I'm going to get my friend to break me out.' I can't tell if she's joking.

To the right of the nurses' station, opposite one of the two payphones, is the TV room. Well, technically, actually, the TV corner. It's a continuation of the corridor, with enough furniture in it to arguably constitute a room. Erratically stocked bookshelves, five rows of plastic chairs three deep and a dust-coated TV mounted onto the wall. Around it, at the allotted, agreed TV times (briefly in the morning, the afternoon and then for a longer stretch at night) listed on the schedule that is stuck onto the walls, sit most of the other patients.

As soon as it's the scheduled hour, we take our seats. All necks, faces, ears, eyes, minds directed up into the corner, through the TV screen, through the cables and wires to a reality happening somewhere other than here. No one speaks. Everyone simply stares up.

CHUNG-CHUNG.

The opening bars of *Law and Order: Special Victims Unit*. The noise that had resonated around every apartment I'd lived in for the last few years. Every day, every night, I'd sought comfort in the dark, in the stories of women who had been pared and pillaged like me. Each episode saw them, faces bruised, bodies smashed, hearts emptied out, getting justice. I would watch episode after episode, my heart hammering every time The Bad Man paid for his Awful Crimes. The victim, the woman, walking straight-backed, proud, resilient into her future. Made whole again by the destruction of the one who'd tried his best to bloody her beyond redemption, to ruin her forever.

The TV shudders on the bracket. It amazes me that this is considered acceptable entertainment for a room full of psychiatric patients. We watch episode after episode: stories of rape, murder, abuse, unimaginable cruelties visited on the weakest, most vulnerable. Everyone sits unflinching, unmoving, as crimes are committed, justice served.

Later, I go to the AA meeting, thinking it'll be one mark in my favour with the doctors. It's held in a small side room opposite the break room. Inside are eight other people from the ward and a woman who's come in from the outside world to tell us her story. I'm the only first-timer in the room and I'm given an information leaflet that I squeeze into a ball in my hands.

The woman from the outside begins talking. There's a small window above her head that looks out onto the street, the sky, a building nearby. The glimpse of the world is intoxicating and my head spins.

She's like me, kind of. She had a good job, friends, but as she drank more and more, she ended up in situations that I'd lived too. Blacking out, upsetting those she loved, falling down the stairs, breaking a bone, almost getting arrested. My teeth start to lightly clatter as my face bristles and throbs in recognition; the voice in my head saying that I don't belong here gets a little quieter. Every excuse I've come up with, every way I've rationalised starts to feel slippery between my fingers. She speaks of how much better her life has become. How happy she is, now that she's committed to the programme and submitted to the higher power.

Others are invited to share their stories. James from the ward starts to talk. He's tall, grey-haired, wears glasses. In his khaki shorts and sandals, you'd take him to be an off-duty estate agent or ad sales guy. He turned up in New York a handful of days ago, running from another city he didn't want to be, or couldn't be, in any more. He had no money, nowhere to stay and just a bagful of clothes. He went to a bar and hooked up with an older man he wasn't attracted to, just so he'd have somewhere to sleep. They stayed up doing pills for a couple of days. It's not clear if it was the drugs or the hook-up that sent him spiralling but he ended up in the emergency room and then here.

His family are down south, but he isn't so welcome after multiple relapses and addictions and arrests. He has nieces and nephews who need to be sheltered and shielded from his behaviour. He nods as he recounts this, while tears fill his eyes. He has spent decades hustling for money, booze, drugs, a roof over his head. Decades being passed around and used, using others. He's been diagnosed as bipolar and medicated for some time, but he always goes back to the drugs he gets off the street; the prescriptions are never enough.

I think of my own niece, the love of my life: what I owe her. How much I don't want to let her down. I keep listening. I don't speak in this session, but I put my hands in the palms of others when everyone stands to say the serenity prayer at the end. *God, grant me the serenity to accept the things I cannot change, courage to change the things I can, And the wisdom to know the difference.* The girl like me smiles and says, 'Keep coming back.'

CHAPTER 26

I t's the next afternoon and TV hour again. I'm seated four rows back. The man in front of me – a grey-haired, middle-class dad – starts to jerk backwards and forwards, the legs of his chair scraping in quick movements along the floor, like a man standing up, pushing his chair back, then changing his mind. Over and over again at speed. It takes me a moment to work out what's happening, until his head snaps back and forth and one of the other patients shouts, 'He's having a fit!'

We call out to the nurses who, for pretty much the first time ever, aren't standing there watching us. They run over and lay him carefully on the floor. We're all sent into the other room, where we try to look through the window, but can't quite see what's happening. Some minutes later, he's wheeled past us, an oxygen mask on his face.

The rumours circulate. *He died, right there on the floor. He had a seizure brought on by ECT* (Electroconvulsive Therapy). *He'd had a stroke. He was in a coma.* When he does return to the ward some days later, his eyes are empty and deep.

He's not the only one undergoing ECT. The hospital, I'm told, are 'bringing it back', advocating it as a course of treatment for depression which doesn't respond to medication in those patients who are the hardest to reach. One patient, a forty-something New Jersey wife and mother, has it every other day. She is bright, funny, sharp. She tells me her husband is something in the mafia, a mob boss. He controlled her for decades. They have two kids. She loves them; he controls them. Their marriage hit trouble; she sank into a deep and ever deeper depression until eventually he found her hanging from the light fitting in their bedroom.

'He didn't call an ambulance.' She laughs. A friend saved her, got her medical attention. In the months since she's been sectioned he's been to see her just a handful of times. She speaks to her kids on the phone but they rarely visit. She's torn as to whether it's for the best. For them, for her. She suspects it's for the best for him.

She is taken off for her treatment in the morning while we're still asleep. As we eat breakfast, her unconscious body is wheeled past the break room. Heads swivel left and right to look as the gurney is wheeled past, wheels creaking. She'll join us a couple of hours later, sore, a little quieter than normal.

One day I ask her: 'Does it hurt?'

'Yes,' she answers. 'They tell you it won't, but it does. But mostly it's the headache afterwards.'

'And do you feel better?'

'No,' she says firmly. 'They told me I had to have it

to even begin the conversation about getting out as I felt just as depressed as I ever have done. But I still feel the same. I tell them I don't so they don't keep me in here forever.'

There's the tall, intimidating brunette, who has a young daughter out in the world and another baby brewing in her belly. Her daughter sometimes comes to visit, her small eyes round and terrified as she clings to the woman who brings her in. The brunette's fuzzy black hair is pulled back into a rough ponytail; she has brown, smudged circles under her dark eyes, tattoos on her arms. She dresses every day in jogging bottoms, pyjamas and vests. She tells me that she's been addicted to drugs, to heroin, and has suffered multiple breakdowns. She's worried about her daughter, having watched her own mother spend almost her entire childhood in a long-term institution in upstate New York. Her childhood memories were of her mum getting hospitalised, being gone for months, then years, coming back for brief periods before needing to go away again. She is painfully, excruciatingly aware of history repeating itself and is determined to do better, be better, get better. This determination is the only possible way I can explain the treatment she is exposing herself to: electric shock therapy while five months pregnant.

'Oh God, how can that possibly be safe?' I gasp at her as she rubs her belly. 'When you get shook, when your bones get shook, doesn't the baby get hurt?'

She shrugs and shakes her head at the same time.

'No, the doctors told me it was perfectly safe.' In here, she is safe from heroin, a drug that has followed her around for years. She's tried everything to leave it behind, over and over. It's impossible to tell where the mental illness ends and her drug addiction begins.

Almost every single person on the unit has a substance abuse issue. Drinks, pills, heroin, meth. I wonder what comes first: the booze, the drugs, or the madness? Do the addictions drive them crazy or are they simply trying to keep the hell at bay by whatever means necessary?

And everyone has their own story to tell. So much worse, it seems, than mine.

The fear is what connects us. The patients from different countries, of different ages, generations, back-grounds, lives outside of here. The fear that we'll stay locked inside for weeks, months, years. Forever. Apart from Daniel.

He doesn't want to go. His life outside is chaotic. Moving between homes of relatives, shelters, the streets. Getting access to his medication and taking care of his mental health is almost an impossibility. In here, he's part of a community. He has a structure, a role. He matters.

At night, the supper trolley is brought out – snacks, sandwiches, fruit and yoghurt to tide us over until morning. And every night, the same thing happens. Louise, the woman I'd sat across from at breakfast on the first morning, who barely speaks a single, solitary word, walks into the break room, strides up to the trolley, takes a tuna-fish sandwich and sticks it down her pants, pulling her drawstring trousers tight over them. She walks around with it tucked in there all night. I can still hear her:

Sway, sway, shuffle, shuffle, rustle, rustle.

Mob Boss Wife shares a room with her and tells me that every night when they go to bed – at least two hours after the arrival of the supper trolley – Louise gets undressed, takes the tuna-fish sandwich out of her knickers, unwraps it and eats it, slowly and methodically, licking each finger as she does.

CHAPTER 27

We hear the screaming before we see where it's come from: the guttural howling ringing out on a loop. Each cycle abruptly halted with a sharp intake, then swallow of breath before it begins again.

We exchange glances across the table – mine as the new girl, unfamiliar with what could have caused the screaming, panicked, searching, looking for answers. Those with a little more time under their belt have a knowing look born of knowledge and experience. They have seen this before. Everyone cranes their necks to look out into the corridor. There, with a member of staff either side, is a thirty-something Asian-American woman, who is currently baring her throat to the ceiling, digging her socked feet into the polished floor in vain. They're pulling her towards the door by the nurses' station that I haven't seen anyone go through yet.

'I'm gonna sue you,' she shouts between screams. 'You are so going to regret this!' She attempts a laugh before screaming again.

'Where are they taking her?' I ask.

'Seclusion,' says Daniel. 'The padded cell.'

Seeing my alarm, he pushes his glasses up his nose and collapses into laughter.

'What?!' I say.

Sarah rolls her eyes, puts a palm on the table and shares what sounds like part-truth, part-horror, part-mythology: 'If someone's not . . . cooperating, or has properly lost it, they get taken to isolation for a day or two.'

Apparently in the room there is no bed frame, no desk, no TV. Just a mattress on the floor. Whoever is in there is on twenty-four-hour watch. A member of staff, sentry-like, sits on a plastic chair in the corner, their back against the wall. They say the walls, the floors, the doors are all white. I think about what it must be like to be inside that bleached, blank room, the proximity of one person whose only job is to watch you. Do you try to make conversation with them, stare past them? I can barely imagine how thin the minutes and hours would become, stretching out for eternity in there.

Apparently, The Screamer will be kept in there until the 'episode' passes.

It passes by the next day, when she pads through the communal space in front of the nurses' station. She's no longer screaming, but she's clearly furious, her jaw hard and square. It's phone hour – the time when friends and family can call one of the two payphones or, if you have a telephone card, you can call them. She waits in line, people eyeing her warily, pretending not to listen, but desperate to hear who she can possibly be calling and what she can be saying. It turns out that she's calling her lawyer. And it's a good lawyer. She's telling him that he needs to get her out, right now.

If you disagree with the hospital's decision to commit you, you're able to appeal their decision. There is a hospital 'courtroom' where cases are heard every few days. I had been told about the process when I asked about my options. I'd also been told that it usually results in people being kept in for longer. It delays everything and also shows the doctors that you are unable or unwilling to accept the reality of your problems and their help. I decided, without much thought, through a fog of fear and panic, that I wouldn't appeal. That I wouldn't fight. I'd be a good girl – a role I knew how to play to a tee – until they decided I could leave.

And in this sense, oddly the rhythm of the hospital suits me. I've always been a good girl. Excelled at it, in fact. I'd been born with, or at least had instilled at an early age, a desire to please, to be given approval and the warmth of attention. People could feel it radiate off me. It gave me a neediness that made my mum's skin itch. I needed her, specifically. She felt it whenever we were in the same room, my eyes, always pleading and hopeful, turned towards her as she did her best to deflect. Men felt it. Saw my need and along with it compliance, if not a willingness to be coerced with ease. They knew part of me would likely be grateful, that calling me 'special' would quell the desire to fight. That being the first person to tell me I was worth something would wrongfoot me enough to blur the lines of what was wrong and what was right and *was this love?*

The days and nights in the hospital are simple and structured in a straight line around one thing and one thing only: being a good girl and getting the fuck out of there. The days always begin the same way: I wake up, though I have never really slept that well – an opened-every-ten-minutes door, writing on clipboards and constant low lights making sleep impossible. The first night I'd woken up pretty much every time the nurse pushed the handle and moved their upper body inside. Startled, fingers gripping the starched sheets, as I remembered once again where I was and what they were doing. They weren't an intruder, leaning in, bringing in danger, violating the safety of my space. They were there to keep the danger out or at least keep it down, tightly locked inside me. Their job was to stop it coming out of me and smothering me as I slept. There were no curtains on the windows, just the wire mesh, which blocked out next to no sunlight. I've accepted this as my new reality, submitted to it with speed and ease.

But this woman isn't. She is fighting. Hard. Rumour on the ward is that she's a high-powered exec in a big tech company. She has a huge job, a six-figure salary and, frankly, they've fucked with the wrong person. Word is that she came in feeling tired and burnt out, signed some forms she hadn't read properly, and before she could say 'court order' found herself being escorted up

208

to the eighth floor. Stories like these are common – the woman who turned up in the emergency room suffering exhaustion, asking for someone to soothe the edges; the one who couldn't sleep and wanted to be helped under. Who'd presented themselves to doctors and nurses on their very last nerve. Who'd been 'tricked, duped', into staying a night or maybe two – for a rest – and were now locked up in here with us, the mad ones, desperate to escape from the prison they'd found themselves in.

Everyone rolls their eyes as she rants and raves on the phone, clearly trying to ensure that her feelings reach the nurses, which may then reach the doctors.

'They'll just keep her in for longer,' say the old hands. 'She'd be better off just doing her three days and getting out.'

In the meantime, with the screaming stopped and her hearing not until tomorrow, she joins us for an art class. We sit around the square table in the art room – which is a room full of supplies nearest the locked double doors. There's a pile of paper in the middle of the table, paints, charcoal, pencils and pens. We're told to paint or draw whatever we feel. I paint a woman with almond eyes, towering bulbous hair and fire and darkness all around her. Her smile is a slash of red. The Screamer is talking softly to Jean, murmuring in her ear, softly drawing. Jean has been in the ward the longest. She's in her sixties, her short grey hair curling at the nape of the neck. She wears sweatpants and a sweater, both grey. When she's not in class, she walks the halls – one end to the other – over and over and over. She doesn't so much walk as shuffle.

The sounds of her slippers move down the polished floor, moving at exactly the same speed and with the same rhythm, for hours. The sound of Jean shuffling soundtracks the day: behind the TV, behind the chatting staff, the patients sparring, is Jean. They say that she's been here for several months, if not years. That either her husband died or left her or she never had one. That she has kids or none. That she only speaks when it's absolutely necessary. When it's necessary is during the colour therapy group.

'What colour are you today?' asks the group leader.

I say I'm red, feeling it's violent and vivid but not anything alarming enough to add on any more days. Jean's next. I wonder if she'll answer at all. I realise that if she does it will be the first time I've heard her voice.

'Jean?' comes the prompt.

'Black,' she says. 'Black.'

My heart breaks. I wonder what has made her so sad. So alone. Where the only life she feels able to live is one where she gets up every morning, showers, puts on the same clothes, puts on her socks, her slippers and shuffles inch by inch, step by step, up and down the hospital hallways. Where she doesn't speak, breathe, utter a word for the majority of her day. Her thoughts, her fears, her regrets, every feeling, every emotion kept inside, under her skin and between her bones. Those things had to snake and swim inside her, in the gaps, but they never came out, she never gave voice to them. I think how lonely she must feel: here and out in the world at large. I try to picture her walking down the street, in Trader Joe's, on the subway, but can only ever see her the same way: shuffling, sliding down the polished floor, hands stiff as boards by her sides.

Later, there's scent class: a clutch of perfumes, of lotions and potions – the point, we're told, is to connect us with our senses. A useful stop on the journey to self they are trying to help us on. We sit crowded around the table, lifting bottle necks and nozzles to our noses to inhale deeply. We have to use words to describe what we smell and how it makes us feel. I pick up a generic bottle and ramble something about 'life' and 'energy' and 'lightness', one eye on the member of staff patrolling the rec room. Because in every class, in every session, is a member of staff, clipboard rested against their gut, scribbling down what each of us are doing.

It's why I get up, dress and join in every day. Not because I think scent class will change me or help me or make the tiniest dent in the madness infesting my mind – but because I want to get out.

Although even I almost say no to chair yoga. '*Chair yoga?*' I ask.

'Yep. So everyone can take part,' says a member of staff.

I walk into the recreation room cum breakfast hall cum meeting room. A handful of the other patients are seated, waiting to start. I take an empty chair, offering weak smiles at my classmates that aren't returned. The instructor starts talking us through simple positions and poses as we all stay seated in our plastic chairs. Everyone's wearing their normal clothes. We sit, some of us panting, raising our arms above our head and then down to the floor in the most unathletic and inauthentic yoga class of all time.

The only one I go to willingly, speed in my step, is music group. Because as well as control over the television, and being able to watch films at the drop of a hat (though it is a stroke of luck that everyone else in the ward, male and female, seems only to want to watch *Law and Order: SVU* and *Criminal Minds* during TV time – they truly are the great unifiers), I desperately miss music. No phone and no computer means no music.

My ears are starved, my heart and mind quiet. When I arrive at the class, there is a woman, the group leader, holding a black boom box, which must have been from the 90s. She has a slipcase book full of loose CDs and a stack in plastic cases, many cracked, the clear plastic now lined and milky. She's passing them around the group, who are regarding them with a mixture of excitement and suspicion. The task at hand: to pick a CD, a song on it, that means something and play it. We're going around in a circle – they choose songs that remind them of school, of kids they've lost, of kids they're barely holding on to, of love they once had. As the songs play, each person leaves the green room, the circle, their place in it, and floats up, up and away, outside, up into the sky where they find their old memories, old lives waiting for them with open arms. With forgiveness. For a moment they're not mad people sitting on plastic chairs in a circle with other mad people. They're real, warm flesh-and-blood men and women with lives, with people who love them, who have once, many times, looked at them with recognition, with respect. Who don't tell them when to eat, how to medicate themselves, don't ask them to pare themselves open like a rotten fruit in front of strangers. They are safe, a different kind of safe. They are normal. Just like everyone else. It's the most glorious three-and-a-half-minute escape from behind the wire and walls. And one that ends almost as it begins. The dying seconds of the song, the fadeouts that they know so well getting quieter and quieter until it's over, the spell broken. Now, once again, they're just a mad person sitting on a plastic chair in a circle with other mad people. They pass to the next person, and their minutes of magic begin now.

When it reaches me, the magic has run dry: I can't cope with everyone regarding me, still the new girl, with such suspicion. I've been fingering the thick black CD booklet, pulling out silver and gold discs and slipping them back inside again. The 90s R&B and Noughties country music is doing nothing to aid my escape. In my head, there's no escape, just a straight path home.

The Jam, taking me home to screaming and broken bones, the warm afternoon I came home from school to be met by Mum on her hands and knees under the ironing board, picking up hundreds and hundreds of shards of black vinyl, now sharp as glass, wincing every time a sliver slid into her skin, drawing a red line as it went, marking its path. She'd been playing a Jam record and her boyfriend had come home from work, thought it reminded her of an unnamed ex and smashed it to pieces and pieces and pieces while she held the spitting iron between them.

To full dancefloors above a village pub of drinkers, bouncing and vibrating to 'A Town Called Malice', swimming in lager and blackcurrant, littered with white crusts, Mum's sticky perm lit right through with disco lights flashing green, blue, red, orange to the beat of the music. The dartboard rocked under the arrows it received and the bass of the disco, coming a few centimetres off the wall with each chorus. The men, all with no hair, round bellies, shiny shoes, shirts done up to the very top. Necks red-raw and slick with sweat beneath the collars that pinched at them no matter how they pulled, becoming damper and tighter as the hours passed and the drinks sank inside and the slick swam thicker and wetter. The next morning the shirt would lie discarded by the radiator, fingerprints taken in the muck, sweat, yeast that lined it, now flaking off onto the carpet.

To a bedroom, the end of a narrow double bed in London, white sheets with creases still visible and itchy red wool blankets tucked in tight, 'Start' playing as we kissed with open mouths and sighed with closed throats, fingers hooked into hair, clinging on for life and pointing towards oblivion, and the room blurring to distortion around us until everything was noise and fuzz and a blanket of beige, until we're submerged entirely. 'Walls Come Tumbling Down' bouncing off the Artexed ceiling of the house, through each doorway and up the stairs, through the net curtains and out of the open windows into the blue sky outside, laying the path that disagreement will ride in on, joined by raised voices and accusations and the creak of barely held tension, breaking like a wave to rush in with screaming and fistfuls of blood, spilling as it comes.

When I look at 'No Diggity' I'm taken nowhere. I'm here, a mad person on a plastic chair in a circle with the other mad people. I envy the escape, the journey of the others. Even those who silently cry, staring at the ceiling or the floor as they do. No one makes a move to comfort them, to hold them. Everyone's stuck in their own stasis. We may as well be in individual plastic pods, experiencing this in total isolation.

The activities room is by the main doors – the doors that are always locked, that allow in the outside world during visiting hours (how it burns to see people come and go freely), but other than that they're activated by a pass or via the intercom on the door. After each visiting session, they lock the doors and the outside world is once again banished.

CHAPTER 28

Jamie is my only friend in town when the overdose happens. My best friend, the one bright and shining wonderful thing about moving to New York, is in LA on a trip. She's the one who insisted I go to the emergency room when I skyped her, crying through the clamping fog of a hangover, to tell her I'd swallowed two bottles of pills. Jamie came to visit me, at my request. I asked her to bring a book, *Drinking: A Love Story*, in a desperate attempt to begin to unpick my relationship with booze. She brings the book; in the front she's written, 'We'll laugh at this over a Martini one day . . .'

It's the most painful reminder that I don't have that many friends in New York. Not real friends. Everyone in New York claims that they're your friend: the person you met at dinner, who's a friend of someone else at the dinner, or the friend of your good friend. The person you met at a work event in the bathroom while washing your hands and who said they liked your dress. The person who never said they liked your hair in the line at the coffee shop, but asked enough questions about it to suggest that maybe they did. The person you worked with for a while in an office full of people you barely recognised as people and you thought seemed human by comparison. The bartender you over-tipped because you were out-of-your-skull drunk, which always makes you more needy and more generous. The person you shared a Twitter exchange with and has 'NYC' in their location and whom you didn't immediately despise and you're pretty sure they didn't despise you either. The British person you definitely wouldn't be friends with at home, but here the fact that you share a passport is catapulted to a top-five compelling reason to be friends. The girl who gives you diet pills from Mexico, because she knows how much you hate yourself and can help with finding new ways to hurt yourself. The guy you went on a terrible date with and it didn't work out but you *absolutely had to stay friends*. Everybody in New York is obsessed with making friends, with collecting them, like the bones a dog will dig up around the neighbour-hood and bring back like treasures, burying them afresh, guarding them possessively even though they never are brought out into the light again.

Every dinner ends with 'Oh my God, we absolutely must meet up' or 'Let's swap numbers' or 'Here's my email', every unexpected meeting with, 'We are going to be BEST friends' and 'I'm so glad you came to New York'. The first few times this happens, I'm surprised that my phone doesn't vibrate or my email ping. Wait. They didn't *mean* it? New York is full of small, insignificant moments that will be carried away in the wind around you. Nothing sticks. Nothing stays. Nothing's solid.

The next morning, I'm off to take part in poetry class. As I leave my room to join the others, the male nurse walks past, the one who has called me The Princess of England since I was admitted.

'Today you look like Fifth Avenue, like Audrey Hepburn,' he says. 'But I ain't mad at you.'

I take this as a compliment and use it to buoy me for the morning, so desperate am I for human warmth. As I start another week on the ward I can feel the despair, the panic, mounting: when will I go home? In two days, two weeks, two months? I know all are possible.

I have my second AA meeting; this one is led by Big John, who towers over the room but shrinks whenever he talks about the pain he's been through. This time, for the first time, I speak. I say, 'My name is Terri and I'm an alcoholic,' though my tongue trips on the words. I feel like such a fake. My stories, though true, feel like fiction. Like I'm weaving a fantastical tale. I can't really have a problem, can I?

My next appointment with the doctor is tomorrow. I spend much of the night on my knees, praying and praying that he'll realise that it's time for me to go home. I get up and am ready in plenty of time for our meeting. I say that *I'm sorry*, that *I'm grateful*, that I will *always be thankful to them for saving me* and that *now was the time for me to go home, didn't they agree?*

The doctor nods lightly, but the words coming out of his mouth are not what I want to hear.

'You seem to be doing well,' he says. 'But we can't get ahead of ourselves, can we? Let's aim for the end of the week.'

He may as well have said never. I try to feel grateful that it is at least this week, but I don't feel grateful, I feel pissed off. Not that I can show it. I say thank you, shake his hand, and am back on the ward in ten minutes, shaking my head, to tell them I'm not getting out today.

There are, though, a clutch of patients being sent home today, including The Screamer and Daniel. The former is over the moon to go home, sitting with her bags packed from the moment she heard the good news. Daniel is subdued and sad. He will have to go back to his life on the streets, his life of homelessness, addiction and mental illness. He talks about trying to get into a hostel, have a safe place to sleep, to live well, and I hope more than anything that he finds these things.

'Would you like to get dinner with me? After you're out?' he asks, and I say yes, knowing it's a date I will never make.

After the leavers have gone, we spend an hour examining Hamlet's monologue. It seems like such a pointless exercise. Half of the patients can't understand it. I'm bubbling over with frustration. Even before Mary, the evangelical Christian who carries a Bible full of Post-it notes in her hands at all times, shouts randomly, aimlessly, at us about scripture and eternal damnation and hell. *You're already there, baby*, I think. *What in hell could be worse than this?*

I have all my hopes on day seven being my release date. If I'm kept in I'll be spending another weekend in here. That, I know, I simply cannot endure. When it arrives, I bother the nurses on reception all morning and they assure me that I will have a meeting with my doctor. Ana has already left, vowing never to return but inviting me for a glass of white wine in her penthouse apartment uptown when I, too, get out.

I give it everything. Pin my hair sedately, tone down the eyeliner and red lipstick. I practise looking calm, collected, unemotional. I've taken my Prozac and beta-blockers every day without complaint, twice a day. Attended every group, made small talk with people who scared me, confused me. I've done every single tiny and big thing asked of me. It is time to be rewarded. And rewarded I am.

The doctor tells me first that he's diagnosed me with major depression and substance-induced mood disorder. He goes on to say how well I've responded to treatment, what an improvement they've seen. That he wants to discharge me but would feel much more comfortable doing so if I were leaving to go straight to rehab for three months of intensive in-patient treatment. His request shocks me, startles me. I flinch at his suggestion, a flush flying up my neck and face, as if a dragon has breathed fire in a line across my body.

'Are you OK?' he asks.

'Yes, of course!' I laugh. 'It's just, and I really appreciate you looking out for me, I have to be back at work – in-patient is really not an option.'

He frowns. 'Oh, well. We want to know that you're taking it seriously – that you're committed to your recovery and your sobriety. You have good insurance and we've found that in-patient treatment has a much better recovery rate.'

I nod and smile, trying not to talk, shout, scream over him. I absolutely cannot be locked up for another three months. I don't know what the legal situation is, right there in that moment, but I know I can't do this.

And here's the rub of the truth: I'm not better. I know I'm not. I haven't spent a day, a night, an hour or a minute in this ward sitting and thinking about what *actually* might be wrong with me, how I can begin to get better. The Prozac I've been taking hasn't made me feel even a little better. The beta-blockers simply make me able to walk around and talk without dissolving into a heaving, weeping panic attack. My focus, for better or worse, has been on getting out of there. Getting back to my life, my job, my existence. However bad it seemed before, no matter how bad it *was* before, it was mine. And if nothing else, being in here has given me a basic desire to go home and live it.

He is right to be suspicious of my miraculous recovery and generic statements about my mental health. Because I am full of shit. But right now, what I still need more than anything is to get out of the hospital and regain my independence, my freedom, my life. So I say to him:

'Honestly, I am *so* committed to my sober life, a life in recovery. This hospital, and particularly you, have made me realise that I do have problems, but with hard work I can overcome them. And I must thank you for that. Because you probably saved my life! And why would I want to give all of that away now?'

He smiles.

'There must be a compromise that doesn't require in-patient treatment?' I try.

He nods; there is. The solution is an agreement to go to AA meetings, coupled with out-patient rehab three times a week at a centre in Manhattan. I agree, quickly and happily. He gives me a number to call for a service called Bridging the Gap. It's for prison inmates and hospital patients leaving incarceration and entering AA. They take you to your first meeting on your first day, ensure you're not pounding shots or shooting up within hours of re-joining the real world. I call, am given my contact for the next day. We're to meet in a diner.

I spend my final night in the hospital with a new roommate. She talks all night, constantly, manically about why she's there, about being accused of trying to murder her boyfriend's mother, a claim that she isn't fully denying, while talking in great detail about how she'd do it and what she'd do to her boyfriend while she was at it. I don't sleep a wink that night. I daren't turn my back to her. Fearing for the first time what someone in

222

this place could do, would do, in the space of ten minutes before the next check.

The next morning, I sit, bleary-eyed, with my packed plastic bag and my dead flowers, terrified to the very last second that the paperwork won't be ready in time or I'll do or say *something* that will make them reverse their decision.

I sit perfectly still, reasoning that if I don't move a muscle, then I can't accidentally mess it up. And it works. I'm given my discharge papers, a Bridging the Gap information leaflet, a book of AA meetings and a rehab booklet. Half a tree to save my life.

I say goodbye to everyone, knowing I will never ever see a single one of them again, and a nurse walks me to the doors, unlocks them for me to pass through. The click of the door unlocking sounds like the most beautiful poetry rolling inside my ears. She points the way to the lift. I say *thank you* and walk towards it as fast as I can without breaking into a run. I don't look back, not once, terrified of what I might see, determined already to carry as little of this out with me as possible.

It doesn't deserve another glance, another snatched look. I climb into the lift, ride it down to the ground floor and stand for a moment on this side of the automatic doors, breathing in the air outside as the doors open and close under my presence. I step forwards.

223

CHAPTER 29

The first afternoon out.

'So, how are you doing?' she asks, the woman who's been assigned to help me on the outside.

'OK,' I say.

What I don't say is that it feels like my skin has been lifted off – not bit by bit, inch by inch, like I'd been trying to do for years, but all of it in one swift movement. Like a magic trick I didn't know was about to be performed. A flash and a puff of smoke distracting from whatever sleight of hand I'd missed.

But OK is pretty much all I can manage with this stranger who I'd hoped – now seeking softness and kindness wherever possible – would have a kind face. Her face was a mixing bowl of hard edges, flat surfaces and shadows. She smiles knowingly. 'Yeah. OK.' She holds my gaze as the silence drifts and I try to match it for as long as possible, worried that to disconnect would be a sign of my weakness, my illness. My inability to handle intimacy, honesty.

I take a gulp of my coffee, grateful to feel the hot,

bitter, sugary burn lift me off my feet momentarily. She tells me these days are the worst, that I've hit my rock bottom and that it can and will only get better from here. That I've saved my own life. That I just need to take each day in isolation, one day at a time. I cling onto her words like a woman with a half-inflated life raft between her thighs, cutting into the softest bit of her skin.

She's taking me to my first AA meeting on the outside, in a church uptown. Chairs pulled into a circle around a circle around a circle. She sits down next to me, and I can feel pairs of eyes land on me as we sit. A question: 'Is there anyone who is here for the first time?' I raise my hand. A nod that I take as permission, invitation to speak.

'Hello,' I say, voice shaking. 'I'm Terri and I'm an alcoholic.'

It still feels like a lie as I say it. An exaggeration at best. It still gets stuck in my throat. But they would say it is my disease talking, so I plough on.

'Two weeks ago today I got drunk until I blacked out, like I normally do. I ended up overdosing on pills given to me for borderline personality disorder that I didn't take.'

Tears hurtle out of my eyes and charge down my cheeks. A few of the other members are exchanging looks, or at least I think they are, but again, my disease is controlling my perception, twisting what I see. What I think I see.

'I woke up with two empty pill bottles; I'd taken both, and before I knew it I'd been committed. Then I spent a week in a psych ward. I got out of the hospital this morning. This is my first AA meeting in the world outside. I'm going back to work tomorrow. I really want to drink but I know I can't. This isn't the first mess I've found myself in because of drinking. I've broken bones, cracked my skull, vomited on myself, wet the bed. I ended up in a police station . . .'

I list my indignities like last week's shopping list. This is the deal, right? I hand over the last soiled shreds of my privacy, dignity, and they give me back happiness and the chance to wake up and not want to die within a handful of seconds.

Even though I've disconnected from the talking, performing part of me, I cry even more, my shoulders shaking. I feel outside of myself and yet consumed by grief, sadness and humiliation. I eventually slow my breathing and the woman leading the group looks at me awkwardly.

'Erm, we're not at the sharing part yet. It's not time for you to speak.'

The room splits in its reaction: group one looks at the floor; group two looks at me with a mixture of sympathy and mortification. Group three, a smaller group, looks away with irritation.

I try to make myself as small as I possibly can in my chair, horrified, replaying every second, every word I just spoke. Minutes when everyone apart from me knew

I was fucking up, but no one knew quite how or when to tell me. I don't speak again.

The speaker for this meeting, a young attractive brunette who'd been the leader of group three comes over to me.

'Hey,' she says, with a hard stare. 'You know, you're not supposed to do that. And I know you're new but the best thing you can do right now is listen.'

I nod, chastened. I can't believe I've been in Outside World AA for all of six hours and have already royally fucked it up.

'Take my number and call me if you need to chat,' she says, with the sound of a woman with a gun barrel nestled in her spine. I take it, save it, and then as soon I'm back out on the street outside, greedily swallowing air, I delete it.

There are a few things you learn when you stop drinking. First, booze is everywhere. Every billboard, every advert on the telly and on the subway; every article, story, song; every film, every TV show, every conversation. The giant glass of vodka, condensation on the glass, hovers over my head, poised to drown me. The glass of wine you pour yourself for that heartfelt conversation, the one for relaxation, the one for grief, the one for joy, the one for sadness. There is a glass for everything.

The second thing you learn is that not being able to artificially improve yourself, your perception of the world, the version of yourself you put out into the world feels impossibly weird. You're raw and naked, like a newborn baby, no longer the chemically enhanced you. Now the startling sensation of air meets thin skin. And there's absolutely nowhere to hide.

Every thought I'd ever had, every fear, every moment of shame and unhappiness, every lie I'd told, every moment I wanted to forget was suddenly laid out like a uniform I didn't want to wear. Each indignity, each horror given its own spot, its own moment to be recognised.

The third thing is just how long the days are. I realise how much time I spent drunk, sleeping, or sleeping off being drunk. I can't believe how many hours are actually in a day. And the nights are the worst: in the daytime there are work and tasks, but at night, when everyone winds down in the only way most people know how, you're left looking at the hours ahead of you, working on your fifth coffee of the day.

I don't want to tell anyone I've stopped drinking and so I try to hide it. We go for a work dinner to a restaurant in Chelsea, the first since I've become sober. I order my soft drinks quietly, resisting the urge to sneak a shot in there. As everyone else gets lightly pissed, I stay stone-cold sober and my anxiety spirals. I'm hyperconscious of everything I say, how buttoned-up I remain when everyone else's shoulders start to sag. How fun I used to be. I leave at the earliest opportunity, knowing I still have a long night ahead. I'm awake until the early hours every evening, staring at the cracks in the ceiling I never noticed before.

I dream of booze; I fantasise about it. I think about how it tastes, how it feels, how it smells, the beauty of the three-drink buzz. I become obsessed with it. I start mainlining Red Bull, clearly not willing to let go of the buzz in one form or another. I clutch the cans in my hands, comforted by how they crinkle and crumple under my fingers.

The friends who know try to be supportive. Some don't understand. 'I'd rather not end up sectioned again and/or choke on my own vomit,' I try to explain on the days that those feel like my only choices.

I try AA repeatedly, even though so much of it goes against everything I believe and feel. Every time it's asked if someone's new, I raise my hand, trying my best to participate, to show up. I flinch at the AA talk, the talking of 'picking up' and 'using' and 'keep coming back' and 'a chronic, progressive disease' – a disease I absolutely had and if I didn't think I had it that was just a sign of my sickness.

I go to one meeting in a tiny room up several flights of stairs near Penn Station on a Friday night, where I'm the youngest person in the room by many years, and a man with twenty-five years' sobriety tells us how he almost killed his family when he drove drunk. I go to one in a church basement downtown on a Saturday night. It's been a tough week, and I cry and cry through the meeting, through the tales and the pain, which sometimes all feels too much, too raw. Three women approach me afterwards, offering up their telephone numbers, telling me to keep coming back. There's one in the Village on a Sunday afternoon, just next door to an Irish bar screaming its booze specials on a board outside; this one's populated by club kids and artists and the stories feature even more ego and selfishness. I take my friend Rachael to one in Brooklyn, an open meeting so I don't have to go alone, and we spend the entire session eye-rolling at the dramatic retellings of one-night-only benders that indicated alcoholism, a few drinks in college equalling a problem for life.

One of the main tenets of AA is admitting to complete and utter powerlessness. Five of the twelve steps mention God. Recovery is impossible without submitting to a 'higher power'.

'Rarely have we seen a person fail who has thoroughly followed our path. Those who do not recover are people who cannot or will not completely give themselves to this simple program, usually men and women who are constitutionally incapable of being honest with themselves. There are such unfortunates. They are not at fault; they seem to have been born that way,' warns the official AA literature ominously.

I can't declare myself given over to a higher power. It isn't even that I don't believe in anything. I do. Ever since I was a little girl seeking safety in the church across the road. I believe that s*omething* exists that is above, bigger. So, it isn't belief that I lack; it's a willingness to declare myself powerless, without any will or self-control or impact on my own life.

Maybe it's abundantly clear to everyone else that I am, in fact, powerless. That I have no hold on anything happening to me, or to anyone around me, but I still can't do it, can't say it. I've always believed that everyone is responsible for their own life, for whatever they get themselves into, and the lengths that you need to go to, to drag yourself out. This demand to admit to a lack of control over my own life feels like a betrayal of everything I am, everything I believe in. A betrayal of my independence.

Instead I make a vow to my niece. The vow is simple: 'I will always be there for you.' How can I fulfil that promise if I oversleep? If I forget to set my alarm? If I miss my plane, my train? If I can't remember? If I dive willingly into the darkness away from you.

The first test: a family party I've flown back to England for. The room hums with lubricated laughter and I so desperately want to join in. To be the fun, carefree one, for a couple of hours at least. To feel light, alive. I start to plan: going to the bar when no one else is there. Saying the 'Red Bull' portion of the sentence far louder than the 'double vodka' bit. As I wait, I become surrounded. There's every chance I will be discovered. I walk away and the edge is dulled.

When the buffet makes its way out, I take my chance. But by the time I get to the bar, a voice inside me is screaming *no*. My mouth begins to move but the empty air around me receives something unexpected. I've listened to the voice; I've walked away.

The question I keep turning over in my palms, to find a satisfactory answer to, is this: am I an alcoholic? On the side of yes: my doctors (any doctors), the people in AA, most Americans I speak to. On the side of no: most Brits I speak to, some of my best friends.

I look up one of those alcoholic checklists – 'Am I An Alcoholic Self-Test! Instant results!' – the ones that allow you to self-diagnose by answering twenty-six simple questions including:

- Have you ever been unable to remember part of the previous evening, even though you didn't pass out?
- When drinking with other people, do you try to have a few extra drinks when others won't know about it?
- Do you sometimes feel uncomfortable if alcohol is not available?
- When you're sober, do you sometimes regret things you did or said while drinking?
- Do you ever feel depressed or anxious before, during or after periods of drinking?

The results are always the same. Congratulations! You're an alcoholic! Well, technically, it says: 'You have a serious level of alcohol use and alcohol-related problems and should seek professional help'.

There is a disclaimer – rubbing up against a report on drug and alcohol deaths – declaring that 'the results of this self-test are not intended to constitute a diagnosis of alcoholism'.

The binary choice is suffocating. I know I have a problem, but the rule is that you only *really* know you have a problem when you admit you're an alcoholic. But I don't think I am. I'm depressed, stitched together with fragments of trauma, desperate to escape what has often been an unbearable reality – even when it looked like everyone else's idea of something much more than bearable – sometimes for a minute, sometimes for an hour, sometimes forever.

A problem, yes. A long-time, long-term problem, yes. Waking up clothed in a house I didn't know, next to a man who wasn't the one who'd handed me another glass in another room just before it all went black. The first morning I woke up lying on a wet mattress, my first thoughts going to the waterproof sheet with a screeching, beeping alarm that would go off when I wet the bed as a child, rendering me too scared to fall asleep.

While I work it out, I try my best to follow the programme but the depression that hurtled me down the rabbit hole in the first place is still peering over the edge. I feel more isolated than ever now I'm not drinking. I try not to go to bars or restaurants, because the temptation is too strong, others' enjoyment of lubrication too infectious. I want a drink probably more than I ever have done in my life but there is one thing more than any other keeping me on the straight and narrow: the rehab centre I must go to three times a week.

When I attend for the first time, I'm given a list of client rules. They are many. From the sensible/reasonable ('no weapons, no violence, don't come high'), to the petty ('no beverages in the elevator, no chewing gum') to the puritanical ('no open tanks, middies, short shorts or skirts, and clothes with drug/alcohol symbols or sexual/lewd references are not permitted').

I'm given a brusque case worker whom I see twice, though the second time they can't remember meeting me the first. Three times a week I leave work early and have three hours of treatment – two different groups for ninety minutes. I'm placed with the 'professionals' group for the first one – those who are high-functioning and in a professional career – and in a general group for the second. I hate both. Every minute. Every word. Everyone knows each other, has been in the programme for some time and supports and advises each other. There's genuine warmth between them. I'm the new person and am constantly told that I have to earn my time. I barely speak in either group and am not expected or asked to. Some weeks neither group leader talks to me even once. I leave each group feeling isolated and ashamed and like a fake.

Each visit comes with a urine test for a tox screen – weeing with the door open so they can be sure it's mine. This is what mainly keeps me clean. The shame of failing and the fear of the consequences.

I have heart-stopping dreams, dark-edged nightmares, of the police coming to my apartment to take me back to the hospital. I know I can't go there again. But when

I do inevitably fall, I fall far, arms open, scrambling for air.

The worst relapse: a Sunday. I've been sober twenty-three days. I'm due to interview an actor in Midtown. Our allotted meeting time comes and goes and I receive a message to say that he's sorry but he got the day wrong and won't be joining me. I've been sitting in the restaurant for an hour, sipping sparkling water. The waiter comes back over as I hang up the phone.

'I'm so sorry,' I say. 'They're not coming.'

'Do you want to stay for a drink?' he asks.

Without even considering my answer, I order a martini. As I watch the bartender make it – cutting and curling the lemon, rolling the glass in ice, mixing the spirits – I think about calling out and cancelling it a hundred times. But I don't; I can't. I'm intoxicated just watching his hands move. I sit completely still and force myself to stay silent. When the waiter brings it over, it's the most beautiful thing I've ever seen in my life. Droplets run down the outside of the glass and before I can change my mind, I'm gulping it down, swallowing it hard.

The first gulp burns, but then the second soothes. The alcohol instantly hits me and my head is flooded with warmth and obscene happiness. I order a second and a third and leave the restaurant hungry for more, only leaving because order number four is what draws concern in a nice restaurant. I walk out into the street, weaving a little now, feeling the sun on my neck, on my back, over every inch of my skin.

I feel like I've been given my superpower back; I'm full of life and hope and optimism. I realise how empty I've felt for the last three weeks. How hollowed out. I flag a cab and head downtown, finding a dive bar on the Lower East Side that people like me can seek refuge in. I order a pint of beer and a whiskey shot. Then, as always, I feel the trickle, the stain of sadness beginning to spread inside, into every bit of me. Reaching up through my bones, infecting my body and my brain, until all of the joy has been drained out and I'm just a black hole.

I call my friend Rachael though I don't know what I say. I think I say I'm in trouble. I might have told her that I want to die again. Because right then and there, I do. Because here I am, back again so soon. Back, peering into the abyss I've climbed out of so many times before.

I'm loaded and lost and can't see or speak properly to tell her where I am, but somehow she still finds me and we're in the back of a yellow cab and she's talking to me and I think I'm crying. She takes me to my apartment and puts me to bed, sitting in the darkness of my living room all night in case I choke on my own vomit. When I wake in the morning, she's gone, but has left a message for me, written on a take-out receipt and sellotaped to a cabinet in the front room. It says simply, 'You are loved', and I cry and cry when I read it. I don't believe it, don't feel it, but the possibility feels like something.

A week later, I do something I've very rarely done in

any city, never mind a foreign one I could be deported from: I order cocaine directly from a dealer. I then go to the liquor store on Avenue A with bullet-proof glass between you and the clerk. I buy the biggest bottle of strong vodka, drink it and take the cocaine on the floor of my bathroom, while methodically plotting how I will die.

Each time I go back to rehab, fail the test and say, 'I relapsed', the group leader sneers and rolls his eyes:

'You actually have to have sober time under your belt to be able to say you relapsed. You just keep using.'

Then he moves on to the next person with a flick of his eye. I feel worthless and ashamed. A nothing. A nobody. I stop going to rehab, stop going to AA.

I decide that I'm not, in fact, an alcoholic. I just want to die. And booze seemed like the quickest, easiest, most efficient way to do it. I remember the nights that I took note of how much it took to kill others who'd drowned in booze and made sure I was poured out the same amount. In the moments before it went black, the resignation and relief would fall. And then rise again when I woke, flinching in the sunlight, still here. *Next time*, I think. *Next time*. I up my amounts, switch to liquor, and still the results are the same.

My wish is for death, and until I wish to live, nothing will change.

CHAPTER 30

Nothing gets better magically overnight. In fact, it gets worse. I'm back working sixteen hours a day – I'd been back at my desk the morning after my discharge – and drinking the rest of the hours away. At first, I think I have it under control, but it soon becomes clear it's anything but.

Six weeks after I stepped foot outside the hospital, I sign a big-name Hollywood actress to guest-edit the magazine. It's a coup and, as ever, I feel a chunk of me restored by managing to pull it off. My self-esteem, my fragile outline, is built around work, and when the call comes – an easy, 'yes, she'd love to do it' – the shape of me throbs in thick black, fat with fleeting happiness. It never stays, but for that moment, it's everything.

I'm invited to meet her in the club she co-owns to discuss the details. Our meeting is not until nine p.m., which leaves a handful of lurking, dangerous hours in which to build my bravery out of booze. I have a couple of drinks before leaving my apartment in the East Village, tying and re-tying the headband that matches my dress. I take a cab uptown, jumping out two blocks away – a short walk to steady my ankles and my jangling, clanging nerves.

I descend the stairs of the club, shoulders back, a slash of red becoming a slapped-on bright smile. I'm there before The Hollywood Actress, but her team offer up drinks and more drinks. I order the strongest thing I can think of. It'll help. The confidence and belief trickles down my throat and blooms warmly in the soil. I know I can do this now.

When she arrives at almost eleven p.m., she's polite and kind and generous. I'm absolutely, beyond hammered. We talk about her club, the city, the magazine, about her kids, my hometown. The room fizzes and fuzzes and the heat and swaying is, I'm sure, just inside me.

Then: nothing.

Around noon, I wake up, check that everything is where it's meant to be – both on my body and my person:

Passport? Check.

Coat? Oh, I wasn't wearing one.

Credit card? Check.

Debit card? Check.

Keys? Check.

Make-up? Check.

Shoes? Hang on. Where are my shoes?

A frantic, frenzied search of the apartment yields nothing. I realise with a slow, cold, dawning horror that they're not here. I quickly come up with a list of scenarios:

1) I left them in the club, walking out barefoot.
2) I took them off in the cab home and just got out without them, barefoot.
3) I took them off in the street, for the few steps from the cab to my apartment. And somehow left them there, by the bins.

It's number two, I reason. I mean: I know I was drunk, but I would never just leave them there in the club, when I was surrounded by people. Right? But I'm terrified that's exactly what I did and play the hypothetical scenario like a memory, over and over in my brain, like a broken tape, looping round and round.

Had The Hollywood Actress noticed how drunk I was? Had her team? I flash back to the frowning face of a designer who worked for her when we were at the bar. Was that a memory? Or had I imagined it? Was her frown at my drinking? At me? Had I said something, anything, that I shouldn't? As ever, now it is just a waiting game. Let the days pass, pray nothing is mentioned to me. And it isn't. The shoes become the latest in my funny stories: 'And I woke up, without my shoes! I mean, who loses their shoes!'

The bodies mount up once more.

Meanwhile, I still think, dream, of the man I left in London. Every trip back to that city is spent looking for him, seeking him out: his words, his feelings, his skin, his bones, his breath. I walk the streets of Soho, down, down, down, the bricks marking time, my path, taking me to him.

We meet, cling to each other, to walls, to limbs and lies we'll repeat over and over: *I love you; I miss you; I can't live without you; we'll be together one day; it'll be worth this pain, the wait, wait, wait.* He tells me he likes the pain and I can't tell him that the pain is still breaking me from the inside out, shattering my rib cage with a violent wind I can't contain, blowing through, pulling me down.

Back at work, the successes mount alongside the bodies that fall at night. I, the magazine, win award after award at ceremonies held at hotels with chandeliers. I get promoted, a pay rise, trips to new cities, more responsibility, more hours, more dinners in restaurants I would never normally be able to afford.

One evening, my boss summons me to dinner in one of those restaurants with a restaurant guy making waves in Manhattan. We arrive at his place downtown and are shown to the best table in the restaurant: centre of the room, slightly to the left, close enough to the kitchen to see the action but not feel or hear it. It's a fairly typical scene: half the room desperate to be noticed, the other half desperate not to notice.

Strong vodka and whiskey cocktails are ordered; wine is poured. The business guy joins our table, a provincial guy playing at being a Real New Yorker. His bright striped shirt is untucked. His suit jacket finishes half an inch from where the rounded edge of shoulder does.

He reeks of money – several hundred dollars' worth of cotton pulled tight across his chest. A fat ring on his thin finger. He buys things; he buys people. But he can't buy cool. And that's where we come in.

We tell him: *your food is great; the restaurant is fabulous; the crowd are wonderful; the drinks are divine.* In truth, the drinks are simply strong enough. As always, my one-meal-a-day diet means I drink more than I eat. With each new round of drinks, one of our table bows out. They don't have my fortitude. There's four of us. Then there's three and then there's two. His wedding ring flashes and winks when it catches the light.

He wants to know what I think. I tell him. Liquor splashes; he orders more. The restaurant empties and closes around us. He doesn't want to go home. He mentions a hotel nearby, getting another drink, but then he's getting a room and I'm walking down a corridor that gets thinner and longer the more I walk. We're in a room; it's small and beige and the bed nearly touches both walls. I'm in the bathroom, orange and kitsch and like nowhere I'd ever want to be. I feel trapped. I'm in a hotel room with a man who's married and don't know how to get out, or how I got in.

I'm bleeding between my legs, but he doesn't notice, or he pretends not to, and as the beige bleeds inside my eyes, he's on top of me and I'm elsewhere, somewhere else, nowhere else.

'Stay,' he says, he asks, afterwards. I'm gagging, my mouth is filling with water and I can't. I say *I need to leave; I need to be gone.* I feel dirty and rotten and evil and excuse myself with one *sorry* and a second *sorry* until I'm in the hall and clutching my body, horrified at what it's done to me, how it's betrayed me.

I'm clinging onto the walls, hard under my hands, as I heave and slap my mouth shut. The receptionist's mouth is moving as I walk past but I can't hear what she's saying. I am spat out onto the streets of downtown, my back against the wall as I begin to mourn who I thought I was. Above me, a man who should be at home lies down in an empty hotel room, preparing to lie again to his wife. When I get home, I take a long, scalding shower, my tears of disgust and self-pity running into the water.

There isn't one specific extraordinarily dark moment that compels me to leave New York. There isn't a third-act epiphany. Though there are moments over the months that follow that are both better and worse. I delete the dating apps, retreat from male touch. I descend back into isolation, sitting in the darkness. When I'm offered a job back in London, the choice is clear: to try to live afresh, anew, or to stay here in my sadness, my silence, harden my edges, straighten out the curves of me to be able to survive in a city that I fear wants to crush me under its weight.

I feel myself start to curdle at New York's touch. I scream at a truck that nearly ploughs into me, when I don't have right of way. A woman in a business suit and sculpted hair calls me a 'cunt' at 7.30 a.m. for not refilling my subway pass fast enough and I don't flinch. I'm sharper, shorter, angrier, less patient, more irritated. I always believed that I would shape New York around me: I was incontrovertibly me and this would be the case wherever I lived. Even in a city as brutal and averse to bargaining as New York. But in the end, of all my complicated affairs, my one with New York is in so many respects the most complicated of all.

When the lust, the longing, the belief that I could be reborn there starts to fade – if it has ever truly been there – the city is hard and cruel. It is the boyfriend from the days before you knew better, who's hotter than you and makes you work your arse off to keep him, suffering a raft of indignities and humiliations along the way. The mornings on your back, the nights on your knees. He might be the love of your life, but you're certainly not his. In fact, he, it, doesn't give a fuck.

The moments are still there. The flashes of cinema and poetry. When I'm hurtling along in a yellow cab as the city lights flash by; when I'm watching a movie under the Brooklyn Bridge as the sun dips slowly behind it; when I'm walking through Times Square, all lit up like a Christmas tree, at three a.m. in July; when I'm nursing a beer on a roof while the skyline dances in the distance. Then, for a few seconds, it feels like pure magic. I rub my eyes and blink hard, convinced that when I open them again it will have disappeared. And yet, in these moments, I feel unreal. The city feels unreal. What do you do when life is a series of beautifully crafted moments but those moments aren't enough to make up a life? And certainly not a life that you can sink back into feeling safe and secure and loved. And *enough*. It's certainly not the city to seek refuge in from the bombs dropping in your head. To fill your gaps, your holes, seal the fractures shut.

On the surface, I am not beautiful enough, pretty enough. I am not thin enough for New York. My hair isn't thick enough. I am not rich enough. My clothes are not expensive enough. But really, it's that I'm too needy for New York. Too raw, too exposed and brittle.

My final week in the city. I'm on the subway; it's a normal Wednesday morning. At Eighth Avenue, a woman gets on, homeless and clearly mentally distressed. She's wearing a dirty vest and jogging bottoms, her hair and eyes wild. She jumps onto the train, shouting as the commuters around her flee up the carriage. As she continues to shout, she starts to tug at her trousers, pulling them down before squatting. We all know in that instant what she's going to do. The carriage splits: those who roll their eyes and sit further away or get off the train entirely and those who laugh, hard, hands shaking while they line up the camera on their phone to get her shitting on the subway train floor in HD. That the subway cars are populated by the homeless, the mentally ill – who aren't medicated, don't even have a doctor or medical insurance – isn't news in New York. Everyone knows it; no one talks about it. They ignore it, they laugh about it.

It's part of the schizophrenic stitching of a city that has two faces. The dance parties on street corners just above the trains speeding through mud and rain puddles, carrying the city's sickest people.

None of this makes it easy to decide to leave the city that everyone tells you will make your dreams manifest. Fear snakes around my guts as the question flashes across my mind: who decides to leave *New York*? I sit on the kerb near my office, debating whether I should stay or go, and a friend poses the question that cuts through all of the noise.

'Why do you want to stay?' he asks.

'Well, what would people say if I didn't?' I shoot back. 'They'd think I was mad.' I know even before the words have travelled through the air that this couldn't, shouldn't be enough to keep me here.

I want more than an envied life. More than an idea of a life, a dream you're sold without looking at the small print. I want somewhere to live, something to love, and I want it to be real.

I want to lay the ghosts to rest, bury their human bodies under the soil once more. This time never to be resurrected.

I want to feel something other than pain and oblivion, fear and dread. I don't want to feel death following me around, the shadow on my back. I want to shake him loose once and for all. Tell him it's different now, *I'm* different now.

I could even, I think, see over the brow of the hill

marked death. Spy what it would look like, be like. Feel enough life stir within me to stay alive. Start to believe that I might look back, over my shoulder, to the barren brown land where I'd just stood. And maybe I'd feel sorry for the person I left behind, when she's both everything and nothing to me.

She is the person I leave far behind on the September day I finally leave New York. As the cab speeds towards JFK, she stays, stuck in the shadows of the city. It was either her or me. And it had to be me.

Sixteen hours later, I wake up in a flat in an ex-council block in Bethnal Green. There is woodchip wallpaper, painted white. No furniture other than a bed, one set of drawers and a sofa. As the sun charges in through the branches that tap against the bedroom window, I feel it hit my face. I smile.

Some nights, in my dreams, I stand stock-still in tight city streets. The buildings, the avenues, the windows are black. Silence surrounds me. I'm screaming at the sky but no noise leaves my mouth; the vapours that leave me collect amongst the clouds, filling the lid over my head. I open my eyes. It was just a dream. And now it's over.

ACKNOWLEDGEMENTS

The process of writing this book, of revisiting the very worst of times, was long and often bruising and something I had to undertake entirely alone. Thank you, Daniel, for providing the space, safety and love for me to do so. I'm sorry for all the times I didn't make it to the pub.

I will always be grateful to New York for gifting me you, Lindsey. You helped me save myself, more than once. Thank God for us (but mainly, thank God for you).

To Phil and Karen for the flowers and every single moment of unconditional support and friendship in the kitchen and beyond. To Mandy and Charli, who kept the faith for the best part of two decades, even when they'd have been entirely forgiven for not doing so.

I can't fully express my gratitude for my agent Anna Pallai – the smartest, funniest and most patient ally I could have hoped for. Without you, there likely wouldn't be a book. And certainly not the exact one I wanted and needed to write.

To the entire big-hearted Canongate family but particularly Anna Frame, Leila Cruickshank and my wonderful editor Hannah Knowles for treating my story with such care and consideration. I've been in the very best of hands.

Pamela and Bob — for a house that was so often a refuge, unfettered access to brilliant bookshelves when I needed them the most and for telling me twenty-four years ago that one day I'd write a book.

To my very good pals Ted and Sali for endless encouragement and telling me just to write the bloody thing.

To Rachael for the scribbled receipt that kept me going.

Dave, I'm still so sorry about your party. Thank you for being such a generous, beautiful human being.

To Katie, Simps, Joely, Caz, Wiggy, Ellie, Chris, Scar, Matt G, Matt W, Dor and Annie — architects of the good times and navigators of the bad.

To my *Empire* family — you guys complete me.
And my actual family: Nana, for making me the woman I am today. I hope you'd be proud. Sue, for being so supportive. But lastly and mostly to Roxanne and Graham, who taught me the meaning of family and love. Who were my reason to get better, to be better.